Paul Johnson was born and raised in Newcastle-under-Lyme and still works in Staffordshire as a civil servant. Emma Johnson was born in Withington and raised in Sale, South Manchester. She works as an export consultant in a market research capacity and speaks Japanese. Emma and Paul live in Winsford, Cheshire, with their two children, Harry and Max. Paul's hobby is listening to vinyl on retro turntables and Emma enjoys performing in local musical theatre productions.

Paul and Emma have enjoyed writing their first book – a labour of love – and hope it will inspire readers to think about organ donation and to share their wishes with their family.

We would like to dedicate this book to our elder son, Harry, for being such a loving and amazing brother to Max.

Emma Johnson and Paul Johnson

GOLDEN HEART

AUSTIN MACAULEY PUBLISHERS™

LONDON • CAMBRIDGE • NEW YORK • SHARJAH

A CIP catalogue record for this title is available from the British Library.

ISBN 9781528939317 (Paperback)
ISBN 9781528969895 (ePub e-book)

www.austinmacauley.com

First Published (2019)
Austin Macauley Publishers Ltd
25 Canada Square
Canary Wharf
London
E14 5LQ

This book is in support of the following charities:

The Sick Children's Trust

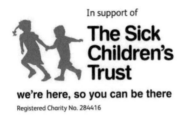

The Children's Heart Unit Fund

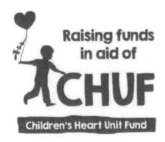

InspiredbyKeira

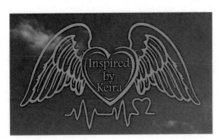

Many thanks to Emma's brother, Marcus Taylor, for the book cover photograph and other photographs featured in this book.

Many thanks to Willow Tree for the Heart of Gold figurine featured on the front cover.

Many thanks to everyone at the Mirror Newspaper Group, especially reporter Jeremy Armstrong for his professionalism, integrity and friendship.

Once upon a Dream

"Once upon a dream, I saw it through the steam
A castle! It was such a frightening scene
Of course I saw it, I had to explore it!
I heard weird clangings and also some bangings
I stepped through the door and this is what I saw…
Rocks flying through the air, all I can do is stare
I knew that sight which gave me a fright
It was caused by demons crying and flying
The air was as heavy as water and around the corner, I saw a boy
He was just exploring too
Together, we walked and together we talked
We walked through the gloom until we saw a tomb
It was so scary
All of a sudden, a massive bang
We sang as we ran to explore and this is the next thing I saw…
A huge hole in the wall
It made us feel so small
In the distance a dragon breathing fire, flying higher and higher"

Max Johnson, aged 9, Newcastle Bridges School – written whilst a
patient at the Freeman Hospital, Newcastle-upon-Tyne

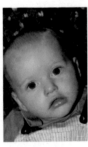

Max as a baby
Photo Credit:
Marcus Taylor

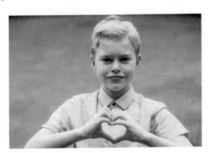

Max transformed by his heart transplant
Photo Credit:
Andy Commins/Mirror Newspaper Group

Foreword

Max Johnson's story is one defined by love. It shines through every page of 'Golden Heart'. There is the love of his parents, Paul and Emma, and his brother Harry. It is steadfast throughout the ordeal of Max's illness, described in compelling detail here, and the seven-month wait for his heart transplant. There is the love of life itself that Max maintained despite the long days, weeks and months trapped on his hospital ward. There is the love, dedication and professionalism of the NHS staff who cared for him. Finally, there is the selfless love of his donor family, the complete strangers who saved his life.

There are many unforgettable elements to this most extraordinary story. Surely, none is more remarkable than the role played by Joe Ball. The devoted dad of four faced the decision to donate his nine-year-old daughter's organs alone. His wife, Loanna, and son, Bradley, had been seriously injured in the car accident which so cruelly claimed nine-year-old Keira's life in July, 2017. He recalled Keira's love of nature, of the animals on her Grandparents' farm in Devon. It was there for 'all God's creatures', from the tiniest insect to her beloved pony, Trojan. It meant Joe knew exactly what his daughter would have wanted; to save and transform lives through organ donation. Her heart was given to Max in a nine-hour operation, filmed for the BBC in a remarkable TV first. Keira donated to three others, including another little boy; her name lives on in the charity 'InspiredbyKeira', set up to help bereaved families, families with sick children and to promote organ donation.

There is raw emotion throughout this book, especially for parents. Joe and Loanna's first encounter with Max, listening to their daughter's heart beating in his chest, is a triumph of the human spirit which defies mere words, and one which will stay with you forever. They are inspirational, as are so many of the key players in 'Golden Heart'.

None more so than little Max himself. Who else has his life story told at the grand old age of 11? When we first met, back in

June of 2017, he was facing a desperate struggle just to survive. My newspaper, the Daily Mirror, had launched a campaign to change the law on organ donation two years earlier. The idea was simple. Around 80 per cent of the population voiced their support for donation when polled. But little more than a third bothered to carry a donor card. A new law – called 'opt out' – would mean everyone would be considered to be an organ donor unless they stated otherwise. It would still be a gift of life.

Emma and Paul had agreed for Max's story to be told to help our campaign. We were put in touch by The Sick Children's Trust, the charity which enabled them to stay at the Freeman Hospital in Newcastle through accommodation which they provide with the help of public donations.

I met Emma in the hospital café close to Max's ward, surrounded by tired doctors, worried loved ones and patients still in their dressing gowns. The pressure of the seven months since Max fell ill with an enlarged heart, its devastating impact, was hard to comprehend. December 6, 2016, was the date he was again taken to his GP. Devastating diagnosis of cardiomyopathy came within days, turning family life 'upside down'. Cold hard statistics quickly followed; 33 per cent of patients get better, 33 per cent need a heart transplant, 33 per cent do not make it. Max's heart was now so big that it was pushing his sternum forward and out of shape. An X-ray revealed it was the size of a rugby ball in his chest cavity. It was a vivid illustration of how badly he needed a new one. The tears flowed as Emma described the 'roller coaster' months of emotional turmoil they had endured.

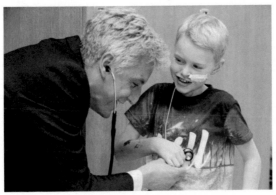

Max with Jeremy Armstrong
Photo Credit: Andy Commins/Mirror Newspaper Group

I met Max for the first time in the play area of the children's heart unit at the Freeman shortly afterwards. Mirror photographer Andy Commins captured Max as he relayed his message to the Prime Minister, Theresa May, on the need for a new organ donation law. "I would say to her, 'Please do that straight away'," he declared. "I would say, 'Thank you so much, Prime Minister, because that would be a really nice thing to do – not just for me, but for other children.'"

Throughout his ordeal – and it is one which many adults would struggle to bear – Max thought of others. Even in his darkest hour of need, he was asking for help not just for him but for the other kids on his ward, and all the other children in his position. When his transplant finally arrived, he thought of the donor and their family, and told me after the operation: "There are no words. I cannot thank them enough. They have saved my life."

As he recovered, Max was again thinking of those who had not been so lucky. Surgeon Asif Hasan was seen in the BBC TV documentary battling to stem the flow of blood after his scalpel 'nicked' an artery during the intricate procedure to put Max's new heart in place. He called on the Government to vote for 'opt out' so there were more organs for his remarkable, life-saving work. The Prime Minister duly announced the reform at the Tory party conference just weeks later. She pledged to call it 'Max's Law' in honour of the Mirror's poster boy for change. Typically, Max remembered Keira, and told how it meant she would never be forgotten. Then, in December 2018, the government announced it would be called 'Max and Keira's Law', with Keira Ball's name added to recognise the selfless sacrifice of donors. It is a fitting tribute to them both and one which Max himself suggested in a TV interview as he recovered from his transplant operation.

'Golden Heart' captures the agony endured by many patients and their families as they await transplant. The new law in his name could help to save countless lives. Yet the crusade for change took years to achieve. It brought some great milestones along the way, and they form the backdrop to this dramatic story. There was the moving speech by Emma at the 2017 Labour Party conference. There was the day in Parliament, February 23, 2018, when MP Geoffrey Robinson saw his private members' bill on the 'opt out' law agreed without opposition. There was the moment when Max met Keira's family so her siblings Katelyn, Keely-Rose and Bradley could take a stethoscope, and listen to their sister's heart.

It is indeed a *Golden Heart*, full of love and compassion as it beat within the chest of Keira. It has saved the life of Max. And it has seen the campaigning 11-year-old and the loving schoolgirl become symbols of hope for thousands of people on the transplant waiting list. As his Mum so rightly said on the day 'Max and Keira's Law' became a reality:

"Good on you, kid."

Jeremy Armstrong

Newcastle, April 2019.

Chapter 1

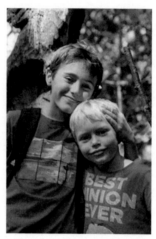

Max and Harry enjoying life before Max fell ill
Photo Credit: Marcus Taylor

"Mum, is it called a 'jewel' carriageway, because it has lots of diamonds in it?" or, "Don't be bossy, like a boot!" or I would say, "I didn't hear a peep from you!"

And Max would reply, "Yes, and usually there are a lot of peeps!" A look in Max's notebook for doodling, revealed a prayer: "Dear God, I love my brother and whole family – thank you for guinea pigs, cats and love you God!" Max's Granny recalls him splashing in a paddling pool in the garden, with shrieks of delight and when his Granny was in hospital once, Max visited her and would make the other patients laugh, by pretending to be a doctor!

Max was a typical, fun-loving eight-year-old boy, when his life force began to visibly fade in the autumn of 2016. He was a little boy who took great pleasure in all that life had to offer. Seemingly mundane observations: "Look Max, a rainbow," as we surveyed the contrasting grey and sunny sky through an invariably grubby car windscreen, would elicit a squeal of delight from Max. Always quite a slight boy, he was a veritable miniature power pack, fully charged with life. With a penchant for walking on his tiptoes, a smile was never far from his face. He would wake up in the morning and practically jump out of bed, excited about the day ahead. Max was always the one encouraging his uncles to 'dust him up'; the time-honoured ritual of uncles mercilessly tickling their nephews. This was in contrast to his elder brother, Harry, who was a far more cerebral boy and most certainly would not be encouraging such unwelcome tomfoolery.

We were just a normal family, with the usual stresses and strains, highs and lows. Trying to strike a healthy work/life balance, but not always succeeding! As parents, we were often tired with all the usual family pressures. Incapable of keeping the house tidy with a perpetual mountain of washing and ironing, too busy at work, not always having the energy to socialise with friends and family. You get the picture. But life was, overall, good and we have some great memories of the boys in their early years. I remember when Max was born and Harry was fascinated with this little creature that had invaded his territory. Harry was two and a half years old when Max took to life's stage. He would inspect and touch Max's toes in awe at their tiny size. Harry went through a phase of feeling a little jealous, as Max was taking up a lot of Emma's time and he would sometimes growl at Max and make him cry. However, this soon passed and as they grew older, they loved their life together – well, most of the time!

As a family, we were never ones for being in crowded areas. We were happy to go off to Arley Hall and Gardens near Northwich, exploring the sunken garden, playing hide and seek, making 'ha-ha' jokes about the 'ha-ha' and having a picnic under the huge old tree. I loved my music and listening to records and Emma, loving singing, was often involved in a local amateur musical theatre show.

We would always try and book at least one week a year in a holiday cottage somewhere in the UK. We liked stress-free holidays, so steered clear of venturing overseas. We just wanted to jump in the car and get there! On our holidays, we would enjoy countryside walks, teashops and country pubs. I remember when Emma turned forty, we spent ten days in Cumbria and ended up practically snowed in. Not surprisingly, the boys loved it and we would trudge through the snow to our favourite destination – the local chocolate factory in Orton – which had a lovely teashop attached. Another favourite place to visit was High Ireby in Cumbria, near Binsey Hill. We always found that part of Cumbria to be less crowded and not such a tourist trap. I remember some years back, the sheer exhaustion and pride we felt in making it to the top of Binsey Hill. The views were spectacular!

In the year or so before he fell ill, Max had developed a real interest in loudspeakers, and in particular mini Bluetooth iterations, of various shapes and sizes. Weekends would, without exception, involve Max using his pocket money to buy one of the small, cheap, light-festooned speakers on eBay, or from the local Argos. Evenings would see him experimenting with various permutations of speaker array, to eke out maximum bass from the assembled miniature drive units; the more, the better. An excited Max would slide down the stairs on the bannister, to ask us to assess his latest effort at audio engineering, a smile on his face from ear to ear.

Max has always been a sociable little boy. Shyness has never been an issue. He is happiest chatting to people – if anyone came to the house to do any work, they could be guaranteed to have a little shadow accompany them during their stay and leave having made a new friend. Even as a baby when we would take Max for pram walks, he would love entertaining people, meaning that such excursions would take forever, as passers-by stopped to be entertained by this charming little human. This sociable, humorous, sparky personality was to be so very important during a year that was to redefine Max's destiny.

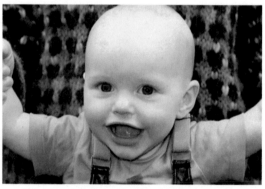

Max – A smiley baby
Photo Credit: Marcus Taylor

It was towards the end of the summer, as the light takes on a reddish golden hue, that we started to notice that Max was not himself. A persistent cough would raise its head with increasing regularity, lasting for several days at a time. This was accompanied by wheezing and occasional gulps of air. A trip to the GP resulted in a diagnosis of asthma and we were duly issued with inhalers of various colours. Whilst these devices appeared to be working a little in the short term, the longer-term view did not offer much by way of improvement. In fact, people that knew Max were also starting to notice that he was not himself; that sparkle was gradually being extinguished by something…but what?

One weekend in September, Max was really struggling. His breathing was shallow and wheezy, and he sat in the back of the car looking so pale and tired. This time, we took him to the drop-in centre at the nearby infirmary. Again, the diagnosis was the same – asthma – however, on this occasion, the doctor noted that Max's heart rate was high, so he was admitted to Leighton Hospital in Crewe.

Several nebuliser treatments brought about a sufficient recovery for Max to be discharged after a couple of days and, whilst his cough did not completely disappear, it was no longer persistent. We managed to fit in a holiday in Cornwall during the October half term, which was lovely, but again, Max displayed very real signs of his failing health. He managed to swim, but remained in the shallow end and would very quickly run out of puff, especially if his head went under the water. A trip to a local castle proved to be too much – he could not keep pace with his Mum and brother as they made it to the top. His brother, Harry, had to give him a piggyback to get him up the castle ramparts. Speaking with Max about this now, he recalls a sensation of numbness in his hands but has no recollection of his brother chivvying him along – his senses were being affected by his augmenting malady.

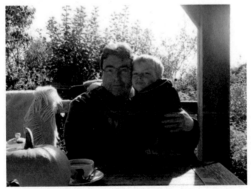

Max with his Dad on holiday in Cornwall – October 2016
Photo Credit: Emma Johnson

A conversation Emma had with his cub leader was again a harbinger of the dark times ahead. They had noticed that Max did not appear to be himself. Normally a very keen outfield player, Max had asked to be the referee during the troop footie match, as it involved less running around. At school, his teacher had also had a chat with him because Max wasn't himself. Max told his teacher that he felt sad that he couldn't run around at cubs or school like he used to. He was slowly starting to slip away from us. We went back to the GP. This time, the doctor thought she could hear a faint heart murmur, when listening on his back. Uncertain of her finding, she asked us to return the following day, when she would be equipped with a more suitable stethoscope. Returning as instructed, the murmur was confirmed; this could be perfectly innocent, as kids can quite often have murmurs, which clear up over time. *Nothing to worry about.* That night, Emma was so concerned about Max's cough, that she slept on the sofa bed in his room and she recalls a very distinct feeling of 'impending doom'.

By now, summer had been replaced by autumn, and the situation with Max was not getting any better. Despite his positivity and determination to get on with life, his illness was placing non-negotiable strictures on his ability to function. Whilst Max did not tell us this at the time, he has since disclosed that he had noticed that things were really not right. Frequent numbness in his hands, pins and needles in his legs and feet at night, difficulty with his eyesight, poor hearing and pains in his chest were starting to make him ask the question, "What is wrong with me?" We were getting increasingly worried and had mentioned the possibility of a referral to a paediatric cardiologist; the identification of a murmur had started ringing some very discordant alarm bells…oh, if only we had known. With the first available appointment to see such a cardiologist being in January of the following year, we began to feel increasingly desperate.

One afternoon, Emma was having her nails done – life was still going on – and Max had tagged along as he sometimes did, but he was somewhat quieter than normal. The beautician commented that Max was 'swallowing' air a lot. Emma looked at him and at that point, she had a very strong, instinctive sense that something was badly wrong.

She took Max straight to the GP and persuaded the receptionist to squeeze Max in. This time, Emma felt a pressing sense of urgency and was more assertive with the doctor. "I feel as though he is deteriorating physically and spiritually!" were her precise words.

"He has lost weight. His clothes are hanging off him. Why is he gulping air? I'm just not convinced this is asthma. Isn't the murmur significant here?" The GP's opinion was that we shouldn't worry about the murmur and that the asthma should be the main focus. That said, she did seem concerned, weighed Max and decided that he should be sent for a chest X-ray. With time to kill before our appointment, we decided to grab a coffee in the nearby town of Northwich, at the bottom of a big hill. We practically had to push Max back up on the return journey to the hospital. An incline that may cause an overweight middle-aged man to break out into a sweat, should be a cinch for a fit eight-year-old. Not for Max – he was really struggling. The chest X-ray lady was lovely and Max engaged in a pleasant conversation with her. X-ray completed, we caught sight of the finished image. Even to the medically untrained eye, the milky white expanse emanating from the middle of Max's chest looked really big.

"Wow," said Max, "is that my heart? It looks huge!"

Emma innocently declared, "I didn't know hearts were that big!" and even joked, "I always knew you had a big heart, Max!" The radiographer said nothing.

Two days later, Max was being sick – not just a bit – large quantities of clear liquid. He was not well enough for school, so spent the day at home. A trip to the local Subway, usually a bit of a treat, was very hard work for Max. He was unable to keep up on the short walk there and back. Inside the establishment, Max was barely able to eat his meal, and that cough...

By the evening, 'that cough' was pretty much constant, so the NHS 111 helpline was called. Within five minutes of the conversation starting, an ambulance had been summoned; the call taker could hear Max coughing away in the background. Within a further five minutes, an ambulance had arrived. Again, the treatment given was for asthma – the shallow breathing, wheezing and coughing all superficially pointing to this being the root cause.

We arrived at the hospital to be greeted by a typically busy accident and emergency department. Max lay on the bed in a partially lit, curtained-off cubicle. Doctors came and asked about his history – had he suffered from asthma for long? As the details of his recent decline were conveyed to the medical professionals, we made mention of his X-ray from a couple of days before. This is where the wonders of modern medicine became manifest for the first of what were to be many occasions; doctors were able to access Max's records and see the X-ray there and then. They disappeared for what seemed like an age, but the doctor returned and, saying very little, informed us that our son was being admitted to the paediatric ward.

Max was wheeled out of accident and emergency, along the corridor which snaked its right-angled way around the hospital, until we arrived at the paediatric ward. We were shown into a bay with two other children in it; a young girl clearly in some discomfort with her digestive system and a little baby who refused to settle, regardless of what his increasingly fraught mother tried to do. Curtains were drawn around bed spaces, but they offered only a physical screen; however hard you tried not to listen in, it was impossible not to hear every word of the conversations taking place behind the curtain wall.

Some hour or so passed. Max had fallen asleep and was lying on top of the bed sheets in the foetal position; bless him, he was exhausted. Looking at him, the sense that he was so small and vulnerable was simply overwhelming. A female paediatrician appeared at the bed space – she introduced herself and then went on to utter words that are seared into memory. "Looking at the X-ray and the information you have provided, it is clear that this has nothing to do with asthma – it's Max's heart. It's enlarged. We think he has a virus, which is attacking his heart."

I felt as though a body blow and an upper cut had landed simultaneously – I was rocked on my feet. Immediately, I made a frightening and ominous connection. Whenever I had heard of people suffering from a virus connected with the heart, the story had always culminated with the same outcome; the person had required a heart transplant. Here, in this paediatric ward at Leighton Hospital on the 8th December, 2016, I had the incomprehensible thought that my eight-year-old son might need a heart transplant. I was numb. I looked at Max and my eyes welled up; even at this early stage of what was to become the longest journey of our lives, I had the gut-wrenching realisation that our time in this world would never be the same again. I just prayed, then and there, that our journey through life would not have to be lived without Max – I got it – our son was fighting for his life.

Emma arrived at the hospital at around half past eight – she had travelled straight to Leighton from London, where she had been working. I explained what the paediatrician had told me and, just as I finished, she appeared and spoke with us both. Max would need to be transferred to a specialist paediatric heart centre; this was beyond the scope of Leighton Hospital. Max remained asleep throughout.

By now, it was getting late, so I left Emma and returned home to Harry. Emma slept – fitfully – on the pulldown bed, next to Max's.

A disturbed night, trying to process what we had been told, passed by; the first of many. Next morning, Harry was dropped at school and I made my way to Leighton Hospital. By this time, Max had been moved to a side room. He seemed to be in reasonable spirits, but he looked tired. I glanced at the monitor, to which he was now attached. His resting pulse – he was lying on his bed – was 145 beats per minute, increasing to 150 with the slightest movement. Even at this early stage, those numbers didn't look right at all.

As the morning came to an end and the afternoon's rapidly failing light replaced it, we were visited by a number of doctors, including the ward's paediatric consultant. We were informed that Max needed to be transferred to, ideally, Alder Hey. However, they were full, so Manchester, Birmingham and even London's Great Ormond Street were under consideration. Telephone calls were being made all of the time. Meanwhile, Max tried to maintain his spirits by watching television and performing the occasional 'dab'. For our part as his worried parents, we pretended to interest ourselves by reading the papers; an increasingly large pile of them was forming on the chair in the corner of Max's cubicle, alongside garishly colourful 'celebrity' magazines.

Shortly after quarter to five, Max got up and left the room to go to the toilet. His Mum was by the nurses' station, finding out the latest situation. As Max approached the senior paediatrician on duty, he collapsed into the doctor's lap. Scooping Max up, he whisked him immediately into the ward's High Dependency Unit (a name with which we would soon become incredibly familiar) and said, "Right, enough is enough; we need to get this sorted." I took one look at Max and for the first time, I properly started to understand the egregious nature of our immediate situation. Max had been placed on oxygen and he could barely keep his eyes open; they were rolling up into his head, as he battled to stay with us.

Within no more than half an hour, we were informed that a Children's Intensive Care Ambulance (run by The North West and North Wales Paediatric Transport Service) would be arriving at Leighton to transport Max – in the rush hour – to Royal Manchester Children's Hospital. I gathered our belongings together, including that enormous pile of newspapers and magazines, and prepared to head home and then on to Manchester. Emma was to accompany Max in the ambulance. She was briefed by one of the ambulance doctors: "Children who present like this can just suddenly fall off their perch." Emma was being forewarned that there was a real possibility that Max might not make it to Manchester, but the considered use of words prevented her from melting down on the spot. At this point, Max was being violently sick and Emma was called into the room to be with him. "He needs his Mummy," she was told. Emma commented that she couldn't understand where all the 'sick' was coming from as he had barely eaten; the doctor gravely replied that it was to do with his lungs.

As Max left the ward with Emma, I headed home to be with Harry and to begin working through the logistical issues a move away from home presented. On the journey to Manchester, Emma had been told that, if they needed to work on Max, they would pull the ambulance over and she should sit in the front passenger seat. Max, for his part, drifted in and out of consciousness, but luckily, he didn't 'fall off his perch'.

Upon arrival in Manchester, Max was taken immediately to the intensive care unit, where he was met by a distinguished consultant paediatric cardiologist, Dr Rahouma, who had delayed joining his colleagues for their Christmas function, so that he could undertake an initial assessment of Max and direct his treatment. It was at this point that we were introduced to ECHO machines. Similar to those which perform ultrasounds during pregnancy, the ECHO machine would appear to be a (very expensive) bread and butter piece of equipment for cardiologists. A grainy image – to the untrained eye at least – appears on a screen; a cross section of the heart. In two dimensions, it can be seen beating and various measurements can be taken, all of which tell the medical team just what the heart is doing and how efficiently it is doing it.

At this point, Max's liver was found to be some eight centimetres swollen, he was holding a significant volume of fluid and his heart appeared dilated. This was the first time we heard about the heart being dilated, but two possibilities were presented as an initial, potential diagnosis. Dilated was added to cardiomyopathy – a word for those interested in the morphology of language if ever there was. On the screen, Max's left ventricle could clearly be seen, presented in the bottom right corner of the monitor as it is viewed. Normally, the ventricle has a shape not dissimilar to that of an Apache chilli. On the screen now, Max's left ventricle appeared more like a golf ball; almost perfectly round and most definitely not an ideal pumping chamber. For the first time, the extent of the damage to this most vital organ could be seen, and the murmur – a faint sound several weeks before – was now described as loud, when listened to from any relevant point on Max's chest and back.

Our cardiologist, already very late for his Christmas party, started to explain his findings to Emma. He stopped. Max was looking up and trying to listen – not much gets under Max's radar, and it would be an unforgivable underestimation of his intelligence to think that he would not appreciate the gravity of what he heard. We would be getting a layman's account and he was old enough to grasp the essential framework of a conversation, even if he didn't completely understand. Moving Emma to a private location, out of Max's earshot, the doctor began his explanation. Getting hold of a scrap of paper, he drew a rudimentary picture of a heart and, underneath, looping between the lower chambers (ventricles) of his heart, he shaded over a line. This line reminded me of the shape of Jack Nicholson's mouth, post his back street plastic surgery, as the Joker in Batman. This was the area affected by whatever it was that was causing this destructive damage.

What he said next, however, was to shake our very foundation. He described the situation thus. Max either had a condition called dilated cardiomyopathy, as mentioned, or a complaint called myocarditis; or both. He stressed that this was an initial assessment, and that further tests would be needed, but the image on the ECHO machine was stark and brutally honest; the distortion and stretching to Max's left ventricle was clear to see, even for the uninitiated. "Children with this condition have a 33% chance of resolving, a 33% chance of needing a heart transplant and a 33% chance of dying."

Here, the words of the consultant confirmed our growing fears, which now crystallised. Further tests would be required to substantiate a diagnosis, but we now had the initial, baseline odds, within which other odds would present as processes and procedures were performed over the coming months. Following the meeting with this caring, gentle doctor, we both sat in the canteen – now closed and quiet, save for the odd noise coming from the cavernous main hall of the hospital – and looked at one another. We felt numb and sick to the pits of our stomachs: Where had we gone wrong? What had we missed? How had this so rapidly become so horribly serious? Poor, poor little Max!

Chapter 2

For Max's first few nights in Manchester, we had a room which is specially reserved for parents who have children in the intensive care unit. It was a very warm and windowless affair, but at least it provided a bed near to Max. The paper-thin walls made it impossible not to hear what was going on in the adjacent bedrooms. Having a gravely ill child places an immense stress on you personally and can test a relationship like little else. In the room next door, a couple would argue for what seemed like hours, after which the television would go on for half an hour before, finally, silence.

It was time to let relatives know what was happening to Maxy. Events had swept us along with such powerful currents, that we had not been able to find the time or inclination to make the calls. That said, love for Max was not exclusively ours – this whole ordeal was to place the burden of stress and worry onto our immediate family and it would be remiss now, not to let them know. We had something to tell them.

I made the call to my father from home. I stood in the kitchen as the phone connected and considered what I would say. It's impossible to know how a conversation like this is going to pan out; up until this time, our emotions had been contained within our immediate, nuclear family. Together, we had begun the process of unpicking not only the medical terminology which gave name to the (probable) illness from which Max was suffering, but also the new and incredibly powerful feelings we were experiencing. Now we were about to share this news with those closest to us, but we did not know how these powerful emotions would evince.

No matter what you do in life, your parents will always occupy that very role and the complex – possibly conflicting – emotions that go with it. Irrespective of what we achieve as adults and what responsibilities we may carry in our own lives and careers, Mum and Dad will always be just that. As I spoke with my father, this reversion to the parent and child relationship started to play out. Maybe I was looking, even at this early stage, for a calming, soothing voice to say that everything will be okay. As I started to

explain that Max was in hospital, with a poorly hea
tsunami of emotion rise up and smash into me. It w
impossible to stop it. As I spoke, my words becam￼
with the crying reflex and tears started to flood dowi
don't want to lose him, Dad…he could die!" Imm
guilty. I was offloading this emotional barrage ont￼
was the first time he had heard of what was happening. So many
times during the ensuing months, one would feel alone as one tried
to come to terms with and deal with what was happening. I knew
that when I put the phone down, my father would be alone whilst
comprehending the gravity of what I had so fitfully told him. My
mother had passed away some ten years before; how I knew that we
were both so desperately wishing she was still with us and would
have this thought many, many times during subsequent months.

We'd lost Mum to cancer in 2007. Whilst she'd had the disease
before, the suddenness of her illness and the ferocity with which the
cancer did its vile work took us by surprise. So many parallels with
what we were now going through. Just before she fell ill, we had
discovered that Max was on his way, but we had waited –
customarily – until the end of the first trimester before telling
anyone. It was during these initial twelve weeks that Mum fell ill
and, ultimately, died. We agonised over whether we should tell her
that we were due to have a baby, but in the end, we decided that we
would share the news. By this time, Mum had been hit with the
ultimate hammer blow; there was nothing that could be done for her.
I have often wondered – in fact, it dominates my thoughts of that
time – what went through her mind as she lay in the hospital bed, in
effect preparing to die. I found myself thinking the same thoughts
about Max, as he lay in his bed; an eight-year-old boy, with what I
thought would be an old person's illness, facing the same outcome
as my Mum.

I leaned over my Mum's bed and, although her eyes were closed,
I knew that she was aware of my presence. I whispered to her that
Emma was expecting a baby, which was due in January of 2008.
Our feelings were so mixed – was this a cruel thing to do? Mum had
doted on her grandchildren – a career teaching children with mental
and physical disability had been the perfect role for one with such
compassion, patience and love. Her grandchildren were the lucky
recipients of this same attention and yet they were to lose this
wonderful influence and Max would never know it for himself.

As I spoke to Mum, she opened her eyes and looked ahead –
"The Lord giveth, the Lord taketh away," she said. How true and

ow devastating. As we sit here now reflecting on Max's illness, ose words have additional, beautiful yet heart-breaking relevance, for at the very kernel of most transplantation is the gift of life to one, at the end of corporeal existence for another. Faith is an incredibly personal thing, but for my Mum and for our family now, it has been an essential element in our survival.

Emma also let her family know and everyone was so upset and concerned. She will never forget hearing her eldest brother Dan's voice choking up on the other end of the phone, as she explained 'the odds'. Emma had let her friends know with this simple Facebook update: 'Our lovely little Max is battling a heart virus in intensive care at the Royal Manchester Children's Hospital. He is in a bad way so please keep him in your thoughts and prayers. Heartbroken! Love, Emma xxxx'. Emma was overwhelmingly touched by the messages of support and love that flooded through. The kind, empathetic words really helped her, especially in those early days, when we were still very much 'in shock'. It is often said that 'at times like this, you know who your friends are'. With only a couple of saddening exceptions, those around us were magnificent. On the Sunday after Max's admission to hospital, I was travelling with Dad into Manchester to be with Max, Harry and Emma. I had informed my work colleagues about the situation, and had received a wonderful, thoughtful response. As I communicated the latest update, a reply landed by return, saying that I was to be signed off work; I could not function properly, whilst my son was in such a terrible predicament.

Wordsworth described the 'nameless acts of kindness and love', which signify the true, everyday goodness in and loving nature of a person, rather than the attention seeking of the grandiose gesture. We were to experience these acts of kindness and love from all quarters during Max's illness. This first text from my colleague lifted a weight from my mind – I didn't feel fully capable of making decisions, so I was truly appreciative of someone making the call on my behalf. Emma's employers were equally caring and flexible.

Doctors managed to get Max to a point of relative clinical stability, whilst they undertook a series of tests to garner a full understanding of his situation. After a few days, Max was moved from the intensive care unit to the cardiology ward, and was tucked into a bay with four beds. As the days passed, we realised that there was not going to be a quick fix, and our thoughts of Max being well enough for school in January were wishful thinking at best. Boy, we were way off the mark. Max had been placed onto a cardiac friendly cocktail of drugs, which included something called Milrinone. This is an ace inhibitor. Now, ace to me means something that is really good or cool. That is not, of course, what it means in this context. It was biology 101, trying to recall the chambers of the heart and what they did and how these drugs, including Milrinone, were going to help. I had roundly failed to distinguish myself as a biologist at school (or any sort of science 'ist' for that matter) and had only really roundly succeeded in becoming, well, round! What the team was going to try to do was wean Max off the intravenous drugs such as Milrinone, and replace them with oral medication. In theory, this would allow him to return home and receive subsequent treatment as an outpatient.

Christmas was fast approaching, and the ward became decorated to the hilt with tinsel and trees and all sorts of festive magic. In addition, we had managed to secure accommodation in Ronald McDonald House, which provides very comfortable rooms for families, so that they can be near to their children. It was humbling, as the big day approached, to see just how much is done for the children who are in hospital, to take their minds off the reality of their predicament. Max met players from Manchester United and Manchester City and was even interviewed by one of the Manchester United players, for the club's Facebook page. As the United star asked Max who his favourite player was, Max quickly looked down at the signed photograph he was holding of his footballing inquisitor, desperately trying to find the printed name; it wasn't there! "It's me, isn't it?" said the footballer.

To which Max replied, "Yes, of course." Goodness knows how he would have managed, had he found the star's name; Zlatan Ibrahimović looks more like a Countdown Conundrum than a name on first viewing. It is telling to look back at the images of Max with the players. He appears so pale and small and, if one looks closely at his monitor, a resting pulse of 144 beats per minute never lets you forget why you are where you are.

Max was gradually weaned off his IV (Intravenous) medication and oral tablets were commenced, which included beta blockers. The effects of Milrinone do not just stop the instant it is switched off – it has an impressive half-life – so the impact of its removal would not be known for several days. For a time, then, Max was free of IV drips, although his lines were kept in. Already, Max had become incredibly brave when doctors wanted to take 'bloods' or needed to insert a cannula into the back of his hand. By the end of his time in hospital, he was able to instruct the medical professionals on where best to go to get the most blood!

On Christmas Day, we were able to leave the ward with Max, without being accompanied by any nurses; it would be July before we could do this again. Max had, as was mentioned earlier, developed a love of speakers, so Christmas and his close proximity birthday in early January saw him expand his collection, but this time he went big! Gone were the small, round eBay bargains – now he had entered the world of KEF and Bose – Loudbox Mini this and Megabox Link that, so that he could hold impromptu discos wherever he went. We took Max to Ronald McDonald and our dear friends, Charlotte and Paul, brought us a scrumptious Christmas dinner. Max managed very well, but his appetite was all but gone and he looked tired. Were these oral drugs actually working?

It didn't take us long to find out. Between Christmas and New Year, Max started to feel unwell again – tiredness, nausea, back pain and becoming breathless were all the symptoms that signed and sealed the diagnosis; Max needed to go back onto Milrinone, because his heart was simply too poorly to cope with anything else. He was now Milrinone dependent and this meant he had to stay in hospital.

You hold onto any hope you can at times like this and I guess that is why the doctors in particular are so careful with their use of language. In the early days, Max's heart function had improved slightly, but let's put this into perspective; it had gone from truly awful to just really awful. However, you pinned your hopes to any visible piece of driftwood, in the honest held and desperate belief that it may keep you afloat until you reach the shore. In this instance, the only buoyancy aid available was the Milrinone and that being the case, we took it without question – never far from the very forefront of our minds, were the odds given to us on that first night in Manchester.

Throughout all of this, Max kept his chin up and the hospital experience proved something of a novelty. Whilst he was undoubtedly aware that he was extremely poorly, the gravity of his condition had not fully landed with him and in reality, it was to be a few weeks before it did. He developed a friendship with a baby and her Mum in the next bed to him. This poor child had serious gastric problems and she had issues with her cranial development. She was a sweet little thing and her cry, far from being the usual, parent-prodding cacophony, was actually quite soothing! This lovely girl's Mum was really kind to Max, and would often produce sweet treats for him...those nameless little acts.

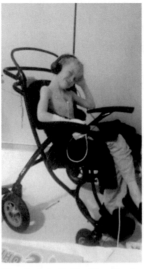

Max in hospital in Manchester
Photo Credit: Emma Johnson

By now, the doctors had a degree of confidence that they knew that Max was suffering from dilated cardiomyopathy, and we were presented with leaflets which explained the disease. As with most conditions, there is a sliding scale of severity. One can function and lead a relatively normal life with dilated cardiomyopathy, but at the other end of the spectrum, the disease can require the sufferer to undergo a heart transplant and, of course, it could be fatal. There was no such thing now as an 'easy read'. What had caused Max's illness was really conjecture – it could have been a virus, or it could have been genetic, which of course opened up the real possibility that it was not confined just to Max, but could be with anyone in the family. At this moment in time, though, due to tests taking an age, we'll call it idiopathic...i.e. we just didn't and still don't know, although the supposition is that Max caught a virus in the September, which dropped to his heart. By the time the virology tests came through some months later, the virus had long since vanished, leaving behind in its wake the cruel destruction of Max's innocent heart.

Talk of the Freeman Hospital in Newcastle-upon-Tyne had featured in our conversations, but they still had a slightly ethereal quality to them. With the failure of the oral medication to break Max's reliance on Milrinone, an outpatients' appointment at some point in the future in Newcastle, was replaced with a more pressing – urgent – need to secure a transfer to the North East. We met with the specialist cardiac nurse, Clair Noctor, who discussed things in more detail. The Japanese have a phrase, 'Kuki o yomu', which translated literally, means 'read the air'. In our conversations with the team in Manchester, it felt like they were very gently preparing us for some big news…they were easing us towards the realisation that Max's heart was beyond repair and that it was, in its current state, not 'fit for purpose'. Max was going to need a new heart. Whilst this was not said directly, the specialist nurse used sensitive language, silence and inference in a way which allowed us to come to the conclusion for ourselves. It was adroitly done. It was not for Manchester to break the news to us – the clinical decision to list for transplant was one for the Freeman in Newcastle to make. Our team in Manchester were using their own considerable experience and professional knowledge, to make sure our feet were planted and we were braced for the news, when it came. We had been battered by the very painful onset of Max's illness, but there were to be many, many more tough times ahead; better you have the opportunity to come to that settled realisation yourselves than have it hit you like a thunderbolt, without warning. Clair also ensured she invested time in Harry, taking him for a hot chocolate and a chat on a number of occasions. She knew only too well that this was having and would continue to have a huge impact on Harry at such a formative stage in his life. Another one of those acts of kindness.

Max has quite a knack at forging relationships with people – a closeness where he can share jokes and pranks and where he can speak honestly. He became very fond of one of the cardiologists, Nadia, who worked on the ward and who took responsibility for Max's day-to-day care. As mentioned before, ECHOs were to become a frequent occurrence to ensure that heart function – whilst clearly not improving – was not degrading further. Max had now been moved to a 'private' room at the side of the ward. He had been suffering from tummy ache and bouts of sickness. Fearing a possible bug, he was moved to a large single occupancy private cubicle with a huge window that looked out into the vast internal atrium of the hospital, allowing Max to 'people-watch' from afar. In reality, the cause of the sickness was more than likely his failing heart, but the space gave him some peace and quiet from the hubbub of the ward bay.

He was now on 0.5 Milrinone; the maximum permitted dose is 0.7. He was enjoying a period of *relative* stability, but this would be punctuated by episodes of breathlessness and sickness. In particular in an evening, he would go quiet and lie on his side. Watching him, you could see his breathing become shallow and fast and he would struggle to get enough oxygen into his system. Occasionally, he would 'gulp' for air, trying to squeeze that little bit more into his squashed lungs. One thing we had noticed was that a bump had formed in the middle of his chest. Viewed from the side, it was quite a significant deformity, emphasised from the middle to the left side of his chest, at its deepest by his sternum. This was caused by his swelling heart, which had quite simply forced his chest out, to secure the additional space it craved. It is ever likely that he was struggling to breathe on occasion – his chest cavity had run out of space and was being deformed by his damaged heart within.

Max's cardiologist was in daily contact with Newcastle, to secure an urgent transfer for Max. Quite understandably, the Freeman has all transferees (sounds like the Premier League!) taken to intensive care upon arrival, where they can be checked, assessed and directed to the most appropriate location for their ongoing treatment. Unfortunately, there were simply no intensive care beds available and Max appeared to be stable. It was clear that the Manchester team wanted to get Max to Newcastle, where he could hopefully receive his definitive treatment. It was apparent that the lack of movement was worrying to the lead cardiologist looking after him. Whilst we were relatively settled with things, Nadia was clearly less so. Never was this more obvious than when she performed an ECHO on Max. The now customary banter between the two of them aside, I could see it in the eyes of this committed professional, just how very anxious she was; her sense of worry and disappointment every time she checked Max's heart was perceptible. By the end of January, almost a month after his move to Newcastle, her fears would be completely vindicated and her judgement spot on. Time was running out for Max – he was in a terminal decline.

On New Year's Eve, Max had a trip to the roof of the hospital with some other patients who were still awake. As 2016 became 2017, they were able to watch the firework displays taking place across the City. 2016 had been the annus horribilis, during which our lives had been turned upside down. I cast my mind back to twelve months before, and remembered that by this time we had been tucked up in bed; whilst the passing of any year has some significance, 2015 into 2016 did not resonate in quite the same way as 2016 becoming 2017. We could state with certainty that 2017 was going to be a tough year, and we found ourselves thinking about what we'd be doing twelve months from now, praying for our annus mirabilis. Parents who go through this sort of experience with a sick child can have a kind of camaraderie; a true understanding of the plight of other parents in the same or similar boat.

On Christmas Day, alongside many other thoughtful gifts, provided by people out of the goodness of their hearts and an empathy for those suffering at such a family-centred time of year, we received a hamper of gifts from a family who had stayed in Ronald McDonald house the previous Christmas. With the hamper was a simple, hand written card, which read 'You are in our thoughts at this difficult time. Take comfort from the fact that a lot can happen in a year, and things will be very different for you this time next year'. We cried as we read the kind words and thought about the family, who had the capacity and love to do such a thing for others going through a similar situation to one they had clearly experienced. What would the next year bring? One thing of which we were sure: 2017 was going to be a defining year for Max and our family. At this time of twinkling tinsel and carols, we just prayed that we could celebrate next Christmas as a family of four, in our own home.

Just as the first week of the New Year came to its damp, cold end, news came that Max was to be transferred to Newcastle. Arrangements were made to transport him to the North East by helicopter. It sounds like fun, but both Max and Emma were very worried about the prospect. It again drove home the shattering reality of just how poorly Max was and how tenuous his grip on life had become. Transportation by helicopter is not the norm, and for pretty obvious reasons. I took a call from Max, as I was getting the car's wiper blades replaced; we were going to be doing a lot of miles, so the car needed to be up to the challenge. Max simply did not want to travel in the helicopter, he was refusing to go and as a result, getting himself into a bit of a pickle. I managed to calm him down, and by the end of the conversation, we had agreed that it could be a bit of an adventure. More importantly, I needed him to look after his Mum, who believe me was far more panic-stricken than he at the prospect of helicopter travel.

One wonderful quality (one of many, I might add) with Max is his ability to think things through and rationalise his feelings, establishing a settled perspective. It speaks of an ultimate maturity, even if the initial reaction betrays his tender years. Before he travelled to Newcastle, it was agreed that one of the cardiologists, along with Emma, would explain why he was making the trip. To be clear, he was going to receive definitive treatment – whatever that constituted – and that part of that treatment would be a heart transplant assessment, as it was thought that Max would probably need a new heart.

It was around 8 o'clock in the evening, when my mobile phone gave its customary 'ping', informing me that I had communications awaiting my attention. I looked at my screen. It was from Max. His text was short, and it read; 'I'm fucked'. The language was not what would normally pass muster, but that didn't matter now. I was deflated – I felt sick to the pit of my stomach and I knew why. If Max gave up, I honestly thought that the situation would become hopeless. I could feel the air being sucked out of me. I had gone with Harry to our neighbour's birthday meal at the local curry house, and I now stood – having left the restaurant as soon as the words in the text had crashed into my consciousness – outside on the pavement. Instantaneously, I felt the very real sensation of loss, there and then. I saw Max not making it, his giving up signing and sealing his fate. That oppressive, suffocating feeling of bereavement; that you will never see that person in front of you again, to touch, to talk to…to be their unconditionally loving parent.

More than that, I felt an overwhelming sense of sadness for Max - please, please let me be able to take his suffering away - this is just not right. Let it be me and not him.

I had to call him – I knew that both Max and Emma, who had been there to witness this poor little boy's reaction – would be in need of support. I was reminded of the poem 'Footprints', at the point where only the one set of footprints appeared in the sand. They belonged to the Lord, carrying the person in need – confirming they had not been abandoned at various nadirs in their life as they had feared. Well, at times like this, families share the carrying burden. At some point along the way, we all had been carried and would need carrying. It was my turn to do the lifting. I called Max. He was scared: "I don't want to do it, Dad…I don't want another heart." How do you begin to soothe a child, faced with such a seemingly abstract concept? How could a child, who has only just turned nine, be expected to react with calm reason? Hell, I would struggle to get my head around this; if anyone should need a new heart, it should be me as the overweight, middle-aged dad – not a slim, previously healthy and energetic child. As his Mum had been trying to do, I sought to reassure Max that nothing had been decided, and that the trip to Newcastle was necessary so that appropriate decisions could be made; "Let's not trouble, trouble, Max, until it troubles us." The reality of the situation was that trouble had taken up residence. Max calmed and I spoke with Emma. We managed to hold it together for Max's sake, but I could tell that this experience had taken another great chunk out of her...our reserves were already running out...soon we would be living on our wits and our wits alone.

An hour later, I was back in the restaurant – I felt guilty, because I can't have been particularly good company for Neil and his guests. I was withdrawn and was deep in my thoughts. My phone rang. It was Max.

"Hi, Dad."

"Hello, love, are you okay?"

"Yeah, I'm fine. Sorry about earlier. Dad, if I need to have a new heart, I'm fine with that. Anyway, this one of mine is no good. I feel sorry for it, but it is no good. I'm fine with having a new heart." I couldn't help it – tears streamed down my cheeks. I looked towards the heavens, trying to comprehend how superlative-deserving that brave boy was. He had clearly been thinking, rationalising – coming to terms – with what he had been told. I was staggered by his resilience. Kids are made more of rubber than the porcelain we often fear. An adult could have been smashed by the news. Max was trying to bounce back. I resolved; if he could be so mature and strong, then we would get through this. His attitude and strength were now carrying me along the beach. Ultimately, the footprints in the sand this night, belonged to Max.

Max never did get his trip in the helicopter. Fog had conspired against an airborne journey, so an ambulance was booked. It was clear that Manchester was not prepared to lose this window of opportunity to get Max to the Freeman, so if the trip needed to be undertaken by road, so be it. Again, Max made the journey with his Mum, who had a similar briefing to the one she'd had on the 9th December. 'Falling off that perch' remained a very real and sickening possibility. For his part, Max was pretty relaxed – well, he had a 'noise' (is this a new collective noun?) of speakers, which were pressed into high wattage service for the drive. Mercifully, the three-hour trip passed without incident and they arrived at the hospital that was to become his new home and where our son's fate – and that of our family – would be decided.

Chapter 3

Max's arrival at the Freeman was a bit of a comic turn. Entry to the hospital can be gained at a number of locations, but the one with which we would become familiar – and which greeted Max and Emma – has two possible entry points. One option is an automatic set of sliding doors, operated by the person wishing to cross the threshold, by pushing an access button. The other is a set of revolving doors. Now, with a stretcher and isochronous machines accompanying a patient such as Max, which option would you choose? A nice set of obliging sliding doors, or the 'mind of their own', variable pace and 'just about big enough for a stretcher' revolving doors? Well, you can guess what happened. For some reason – or distinct lack of – the decision was made to go through the revolving doors of doom…the ambulance crew obviously fancied a challenge. If I ask you to think of The Chuckle Brothers, you'll get the idea…'to you'…'to me'…'to you'…'to me'. Apart from nearly losing an arm, a bemused Max eventually made it safely into the hospital.

In the Paediatric Intensive Care Unit – PICU – Max was settled into a cubicle. The next time he would be resident in one of these would be after his heart transplant. He set his speakers up and proceeded to hold an impromptu disco; Max would now forever be associated, by everyone he came into contact with at the hospital, with his love of music and speakers. Naturally, the doctors wanted to commence their tests, doubtless confirming what they had been told by Manchester, and to decide what move to make next. Emma and Max were met by a lovely Spanish cardiologist called Andreas, who wheeled that bread and butter item – the ECHO machine – into Max's cubicle. At the Freeman, the machines have been given names reflecting a Star Wars theme; Darth Vader, Chewbacca and Princess Leia are no longer fighting in a galaxy far, far away – they are ECHO machines at the Freeman Hospital.

Max's ECHO was conducted in silence, the cardiologist concentrating on getting the data he needed to offer an assessment. What was said here and at this hospital would inform everything to come. "The heart function is terrible" was the verdict. Andreas, whose kindness and good humour we came to see many times over the following months, spoke with frankness and honesty. Whilst it came as no surprise, it is still a shock to hear the reality you face. Unfortunately, how else can it be done? We all are perhaps guilty of telling the odd white lie in response to a question, to spare feelings. This is not something you can do when you are talking about the viability of someone's life. Whilst the truth can be utterly devastating, it has to stand in this sort of environment. Anything…anything which offers false hope must be avoided. So, now we had it from our destination venue; the function of Max's heart was terrible. What needed to be done next, was to decide how it would be treated.

Max completed his night in PICU without incident, but he had established his place as DJ in residence. The following day, he was moved downstairs into the High Dependency Unit – a ward of six bed spaces, providing care for those children who, whilst not quite requiring intensive care, are not strong enough to be housed on the normal ward. En route down from PICU, Max held one of his many speakers to his ear, nodding in time to the beat. Quirky, cute and amusing it may have been, but it also illustrated with heart-wrenching poignancy that, at this point in time, Max did not truly grasp the magnitudinous, grave nature of his situation. In fairness though, maybe it still hadn't *truly* sunk in with us.

From the start of Max's period of residence at the Freeman, we were fortunate enough to be offered accommodation in Scott House. Provided by the charity, The Sick Children's Trust, Scott House is a veritable home from home, offering extremely comfortable facilities, right on the doorstep of the hospital. It also helped that the staff, led at the time by Andrew Leadbitter, were so friendly and always lent a sympathetic ear. As we were to learn through sharply pointed experience, being close by was not only convenient – it was an absolute necessity.

Upon entering the hospital, one is greeted by a modern reception hall, not dissimilar to a departure lounge at an airport. What ends this similarity is that, instead of suitcases, most of the people wandering around are attached to various drips and their associated portable equipment. To the right, as you make your way deeper into this cavernous reception area, is situated a shop, selling stationery, snacks, light bites as well as tea and coffee. A pit stop at this facility, en voyage to the ward, would become part of the daily routine. It was always something to look forward to and it was here that we were introduced to 'chocolate sprinkles' on our cappuccinos...but for maximum effect, this has to be uttered with a Geordie accent. Not the dull "Do you want chocolate with that?", oh no..."Would you like chocolate sprinkles?" is not only a jolly civilised concept, offering a hint of magic in chocolate form; it sounds lovely when spoken by the female assistants in their – oh so distinctive – Geordie lilt!

Armed with (invariably, in my case) a latte and pain au chocolate – a terrible start to a daily diet that only became more imbalanced as the day progressed – a quick dog leg saw you entering the old part of the hospital and quite possibly the longest corridor ever conceived by man; the Magnolia Mile. Redolent of the Green Mile, where the condemned would take their last, manacled, heavy-footed walk to oblivion, the Magnolia Mile – with its seemingly endless creamy magnolia walls – had a similar effect on me. It ran like a spine along the back of the hospital, from coccyx to cranium, it really did feel like a mile. Dotted along its length were doors, leading to dimly lit, faceless corridors, that spread out like secondary and tertiary bronchus. At points along this homage to magnolia, were pull-down seats, or base camps, as I liked to call them. As the months passed and Max's condition fluctuated, this corridor, with its unheard cries of 'dead man coming through' became harder to traverse; my footsteps, like my heart, becoming heavy with the weight of the situation...and possibly all those lattes. Its length and increasing heat as you neared the ward acted as a metaphor for our plight. Corridors leading off the Magnolia Mile offered different directions of travel, it felt like we could be forced down one of them at any time; I just prayed that we were not prematurely banished down one of these alternative routes and out of the hospital, without our little boy.

As you neared the end of the Magnolia Mile, you turned left and, a short distance later either left for the stairs to PICU, or right onto Ward 23. In front of you, as you made your choice, was a charity shop run by the Children's Heart Unit Fund (CHUF). On several occasions during his stay and when he was well enough and free from various bugs, Max was 'employed' as a shop assistant on the till. It was a good move on the part of CHUF, as profits during his stints spiked! On our walks, it was rare that Max would make it past the shop without requesting a stop so that he could inspect their wares. Favourite purchases included Refreshers and Jelly Tots. On one occasion, he bought Emma a hand-made bracelet with his pocket money. One could also purchase all manner of beverages, but the range stretched as far as the latest craze for fidget spinners, with the little circular bearing toys coming in all the colours of the rainbow.

Max spent most of his time whilst at the Freeman in the High Dependency Unit. This was the first treatment space you came to, upon being granted entry to the ward. Out of the six beds on the unit, it would be quicker to tell you the one that Max did not occupy during his stay – the one directly in front of you as you entered. He started in the bed space in the far left corner, but probably spent the longest period in the corner by the window to the right as you crossed the threshold, with a view out onto the grass outside and the large beech tree. Max would often spend long periods looking out at this tree, which he named the 'Tree of Life', in pensive mood lost in his thoughts, the sadness in his eyes betraying a longing to just be able to go outside like other children. On one occasion, a nurse caught him looking out of the window and saw that he was crying. She asked him what was wrong, and he said, "I hope that I'll be able to go outside again one day." It is the crushing realisation that the one you love so unconditionally is suffering – not just physically, but spiritually as well – that can make the whole experience so much harder to bear.

Life developed a somewhat dysfunctional routine, punctuated by periods where the chronic stress of the situation was exacerbated by a dip in Max's condition. As a general rule, mornings would start early – around five o'clock. I would wake and almost immediately, my foot would start drumming the bed and my thoughts would ignite in full technicolour. It was instant. I would think to myself, *Well, the phone hasn't rung yet*, but my attention would then turn to what the day ahead would hold; how would Max be? During the darker days – both literally and metaphorically – the drumming foot would be accompanied by an instantaneous knot in the stomach. A look outside the blackout-lined curtains confirmed that the night retained its grip of the skies, the lights of the multi storey carpark still working to maximum effect. Try as I might, I could not recapture sleep; I was done for the night and five and a half hours was my lot. I would lie in bed, churning in mind and body until I relented and got up.

Breakfast was eaten not out of a desire to eat – to break the fast of the night – but because it anchored the commencement of the routine. As time passed, Max managed to accrue a 'PC World' of new technology; Kindles, iPods and yes, speakers, partly as Christmas and birthday gifts, and partly as a result of other people's generosity as they made the trip to visit him. One such thoughtful act saw Max acquire an unwanted smart phone. This he used in a variety of ways, from game playing, surfing, Skyping and – this is a revelation – to make and receive phone calls. In a morning, I would call his number as I set off for my trip along the Magnolia Mile, to see how he was. For me this was, hopefully, going to be a nerve-settling call.

"Hi, Maxy, how are you?"

"Fine, thanks." Thank goodness! This meant a steady night and a feeling of relative comfort and stability. If the response was, "Not so good," or he didn't answer, then the knot in my stomach would tighten, and those steps along The Mile would be especially plumbiferous. In many ways, it would have been just as easy to get to the ward and see for myself how he was, but this need to know – this need to be able to reassure myself – had to be satiated at the earliest opportunity.

Latte and pain au chocolate in hand, the journey towards the ward commenced. Every few days and due to significant expenditure on caffeine, a free coffee would be offered by the coffee house, in recognition of one's repeat, highly valued custom. In my case, a large latte would be ordered, containing sufficient calories to power me through the day – to add to the year's supply I already had around my midriff. Arrival on the ward allowed me to catch my first glimpse, through the louver blinds, of Max in his bed space, as I religiously washed my hands. Again, seeking that reassurance I so needed. Lying on his bed in his pyjama bottoms and with his hair unkempt from a night of tossing, turning and two-hourly observations (blood pressure etc.), Max would be in need of sprucing up, ahead of the ward round and the arrival of his dedicated teacher, Helen. When he was able and his spirits permitted, we would head to the bathroom to commence the makeover. Max, still with a bare chest, (which as time progressed picked up scars and dressings which left those observing this little chap in no doubt as to the gravity of his situation and personal suffering) would stride – on his tiptoes – across HDU and into the bathroom. Once inside, he would either wash or shower, making sure that he kept his dressings clean, especially – once it had been fitted – the one covering the hole in his abdomen, through which his Left Ventricular Assist Device (LVAD) received its power and instruction from its little plastic clad brain in a box. Invariably, one of his 'mega box boomster' speakers would accompany us into the bathroom, playing whatever hit was top of Max's chart at the time.

When he was on his best form, Max would apply a small coat of wax to his hair, looking in the mirror whilst standing on the little red plastic chair, which was there in case he became tired and needed to sit down. "What would happen if I jumped off this chair Dad?" he would ask.

"Don't even think about it," was my reply. Always late for the arrival of his teacher, due to excessive faffing and spending too long in the shower, Max would emerge with slicked hair and tiptoe his way back to his bed space, pushing his drip stand purposefully along in front of him, pranking the nurses at every available opportunity.

Ward round would usually coincide – just about – with Max's school lesson. It just had to, didn't it? The doctors on duty – usually accompanied by the sister – would make their way over with the ward trolley containing the patient's notes and a computer, and start to scan the nurses' chart at the end of Max's bed, for data from the previous 24 hours. Information such as heart rate (always high in Max's case), blood pressure and breathing rate, would be examined in conjunction with urine output and bowel movements; the latter of which had a number of pictorial guides to assist with a fully comprehensive and accurate assessment of the current working state of the patient's bowels.

"How was your poo, Max?"

"Solid to start with, but a bit runny at the end…"

"Mmm, let me check – yes, that's a number 4 on the chart." Gripping stuff…quite literally, according to Barbara, who had to clean the loo! Conversations with the doctors and consultants primarily centred on Max and were thus usually framed by seriousness. As we became part of the fixtures and fittings of Ward 23, we got to know the support team, which keeps the ward running. Barbara was at the heart of this team. A lovely lady, whose greeting in a morning offered so much more than the simple words she uttered. They had a reassuring tone, reminiscent of meeting that favourite aunt; uncomplicated and warm, somehow engaging you in a welcome distraction from the serious business of the looming ward round. Every hospital ward should have a Barbara – they play a more important role in the lives of their patients than they would humbly acknowledge. Thank you, Barbara.

Without fail, a search would then be launched, to locate the stethoscope assigned to Max's bed space, which was usually draped somewhere over the enormous 'Drager' equipment holder/power supply/lights/bedside cabinet etc., which straddled Max's bed. This mega structure was like one of those enormous cranes you find at shipping ports used for lifting containers off ships and lowering them onto the waiting lorries. Every day, we would be asked how we had found Max to be – he is our son and we know him better than anyone. This simple, opening question was typical of the collaborative approach taken by the medical team responsible for Max. Depressingly, I always felt my answers inadequate – doctors and consultants are such clever people, dealing in meaningful observation – so my slightly panicked "Yeah, he seems okay today, thank you" just seemed to be lacking and was probably more a case of wishful thinking on my part, rather than an accurately observed and appropriately assessed input of real value. Max would then be examined with a gentle prodding of the area around his tummy and liver, followed by a listen to his chest and back. I would always tune in carefully to any numbers quoted, especially in relation to how swollen his liver was. Whilst a little knowledge is indubitably dangerous in this sort of situation, the bigger the number in centimetres used to describe the liver, the more I worried. I didn't know why it was bad, but knew that an increase was not to be welcomed.

At the end of the examination, as Max sat himself up, resumed his lesson or commenced some screen time, the doctors would huddle and discuss what next. Always at the end, the doctor, registrar or consultant would inform us of what had been said and what the plan was for the coming twenty-four hours. We were always invited to ask questions or comment. Quite often, a blood test result had been returned, which suggested a deficiency in some vital element, so we were notified of the proposed treatment to put this right. Never once did I feel in any way excluded from this process, or my opinion undervalued, which to the parent of a gravely ill child is very important. Here was the reality. A look at the notes at the end of Max's bed spelled it out in simple, honest language; Max had end stage heart failure…end stage…we were at the buffers with nowhere else to go. Urgently listed for cardiac transplant, Milrinone and Dobutamine dependent and LVAD fitted. It is a testament to this detailed, fastidious and inclusive care that we were able to develop anything like a routine. There were a number of occasions where, had it not been for the timely, considered and surgically world leading interventions of the team, we would have lost Max in the time it took his poorly, broken heart to simply stop beating.

Being the parent of a very sick child can be a lonely, isolating experience. Emma and I split our time between our home in

Cheshire with our other son, Harry, and being at Max's bedside in Newcastle. We would spend half a week with Max at our second home, before swapping over. If timings permitted, we would arrange to meet at Wetherby Services, which has access from both north and southbound carriageways on the A1 (M). Finding a quiet seat in the adjacent hotel, we would buy a coffee and procure a Gregg's chicken and mushroom slice. Conversation would be wrapped by a gnawing tiredness, but the inevitable discussion topic was Max and how he was doing; a handover briefing of sorts. We would try to keep the mood light by recounting funny things Max had said and done, and always ended by encouraging one another by affirming our belief that Max would get his little gift soon. A kiss and a hug would be our parting gesture and we would then head off in opposite directions. Some people have conceived children in exotic places and subsequently named the child after the venue; Paris, Brooklyn, Venice… Wetherby doesn't have quite the same cache and in any case, we were too knackered to think about any intercrural contact!

Days spent at a bedside could be long and draining. Trying to get Max to eat when it was patently obvious he had little or no appetite was exhausting. His weight was a real issue – he needed to be heavy enough and strong enough to make it through the surgery when he had his new heart. If his weight dropped too low and his strength waned, then his very place on the transplant list could be in jeopardy. Activities were gentle, but it was important to keep his mind occupied to buoy his spirits. Max became an expert at 'Uno', the card game, although his methods on occasion were a clear distortion of the rules beyond recognition. Being on a ward can feel like being in a pressure cooker at full tilt. Luckily, there were play specialists and clown doctors who were there to support the tired parents, who were perhaps either all out of ideas on how to keep their child entertained, or were otherwise too emotionally broken.

Keeping children physically, mentally and spiritually active is clearly essential to get them through their time in hospital. Due to the nature of the illnesses treated at the Freeman, stays are frequently measured in months. The play specialists – funded by CHUF – would come into the ward in a morning and ask Max what he had planned. Sometimes, Max's response would clearly be underwhelming to them, so they adopted a non-negotiable approach, neatly sugar-coated in the form of a choice, which guaranteed his engagement with them. Jo, Vikki, Karen and Louise had seen it all before, and knew just what was needed to get recalcitrant children on side. Magicians, ballet dancers, clown doctors and a veritable smorgasbord of performers were booked to come and entertain the children, but the role of the play specialist was not just for the day-to-day fun activities in the playroom or ward; they also helped out when children went for surgery.

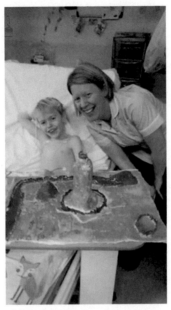

Max with Play Specialist, Karen
Photo Credit: Emma Johnson

Within such a unique department, there are many individuals with their 'specialisms' involved in the care of the patients – it is a truly multi-disciplinary approach, which engages the family as much as the patient. Illnesses such as Max's are real knife-edge affairs, where the outcome is uncertain from one day to the next. What was devastatingly clear with Max was that he was in a terminal decline; his only hope of long-term survival was a heart transplant. Both Manchester and Newcastle had tried to wean him off his Milrinone dependency, but the result was the same in both cases; it resoundingly failed. I have tried to give an insight into the daily routine for Max, but the reality is that his condition made it hard to pin down any one modus operandi for any extended period of time. When he was first admitted to hospital in the December of 2016, his decline was precipitous; without the rapid medical intervention he received, he was very close to certain death. This treatment prevented his reaching terminal velocity on his dive to oblivion. Over the coming months, deteriorations in his condition required further interventions; the LVAD, changes in drugs, increased quantities of certain drugs and intensive focus on diet and physiotherapy to name but a few. In effect, he was like a glider. Leighton and Manchester had caught him and set him on a level course; Newcastle had to keep him airborne until he received his little gift. On very distinct occasions, a downdraft would hit, requiring a change of course to catch a therm, which would do enough to keep him going. However, there was no denying the ultimate look of the trajectory; he was falling from the sky, albeit relatively gently, but time was nevertheless running out.

Downdrafts were events which took great chunks out of your resolve – your ability to fight on – they were a painfully sharp, shattering reminder of just how finely balanced things were. When Max had arrived at the Freeman, they had decided to give it one more go to relieve him of his need for Milrinone. As this was being explained to us, the paediatric cardiologist told us that it wouldn't work, but that they would at least try. This seemed somewhat contradictory and you wonder why bother? What's the point? Well, here it is; transplantation is a last resort – everything will be done to try and work with the organ with which you entered the world. Transplantation is the option when there is no option. Please don't view that as a complete and damning assessment of transplantation; the alternative to it is far, far worse, but there are facts that have to be faced up to.

It was mid-afternoon when the transplant consultant came to see us. We had spent the day with Max, but had been told to expect the meeting to take place at some point during the afternoon. We made our way, in silence, to a room tucked around the corner at the end of the ward.

Sitting on the turquoise vinyl seats, we started to listen to the transplant consultant, a lady by the name of Dr Zdenka Reinhardt. Even at what was our first meeting, one could appreciate her fierce intellect. Whilst she spoke with honesty and frankness, her eyes were full of compassion and kindness; rooted in a realisation and understanding that her words were hitting us with devastating force. After all, she had done this many, many times before. So, why is transplantation a last resort? Well, we were told of Max's increased risk of certain types of cancer, the risks of renal failure, rejection of the transplanted organ, his arteries becoming blocked prematurely and that, ultimately, it was not a cure but in reality more of a palliative treatment. Emma and I looked at one another, and Emma burst into tears. We had just been presented with our new best-case scenario – our lives were changed forever. Dr Reinhardt added that it was a lifelong commitment, and that not everyone could cope with the pressures and demands of living with a transplanted child. Immediately, I was resolved to do it no matter what and so was Emma, but the grief we were feeling for our son and the lives we had known was like a weight dragging our souls to the bottom of a very deep, dark and cold place.

Our conversation did turn to the positives, mind; some one hundred and fifty plus children, having been transplanted, living their lives to the full; carpe diem (Seize the Day) incarnate. During our months at the Freeman, we had met parents and recipients of heart transplants and we were able to listen to their stories, taking comfort from the shared experience. One evening, I attended an event in the centre of Newcastle, where the future of heart services for children was being discussed. In an unusual thrust of bravery, I had asked a question of the civil servants on the stage, during which I briefly outlined our circumstances. At the end of the evening, someone called across the room to me. I turned and saw a man standing looking over at me – he had to be six foot three and was well built. I walked over to him and introduced myself. He said, "I hope your lad gets his heart transplant soon – I had mine twenty-eight years ago at the Freeman." Well, I couldn't believe it – he looked so well – and I found out that he was married with children. As if the encounter could not get any more inspiring, a lady walked up and introduced herself…and hit me with the fact that she'd had her transplant thirty years before, again at the Freeman. It is for moments like this that you maintain your faith in the life-affirming things that can happen with transplantation; that clearly do happen. Google can be a damnable thing – cold, black and white statistics need informed explanation and proper, contextualised understanding, otherwise they can drive you to the very pit of despair. Here I was seeing what could happen – and it wasn't the only time, either. No, why could this not be Max? Why not? If nothing else, a new heart buys him time. The people I met that night had gone on to forge a life for themselves and goodness me, they were giving it sixty seconds worth of distance run; priceless.

So it was that Max was listed for urgent transplantation in the middle of January, 2017. Now the wait was on and it was down to the skilled professionals at the Freeman and us as his parents, to make sure that he was ready when his little gift of life arrived. It was not long, however, before this readiness was severely challenged.

As it neared the end of January, Emma was starting to find it increasingly difficult to answer all the text messages from friends and wider family: 'How's Max? How are you?' It was just impossible and so time-consuming and repetitive to try and answer every single one. She had found out about a virtual visiting room (now defunct) called Just Visiting – www.justvisiting.com – which allowed a secure way of updating, without anyone being able to 'share' such personal posts. She started writing a diary of each week's events, which, although the initial purpose had been to reduce all the queries by text, also ended up as being cathartic and a psychological bolster. Friends' responses were hugely supportive and gave Emma a lot of strength, so we have included a selection in this book. These friends and wider family reminded Emma of championing spectators, willing us on to overcome obstacles, win the race and cross that finish line. Emma often says that she might not have coped without that support.

This is Emma's first entry in her weekly diary:

DIARY OF A HEART MUM: First Weekly Update – Sunday, 22 January 2017.

This week has been up and down. Difficult, but also a relief to sign the heart transplant consent forms on Wednesday. It's good to know we have a plan. The list of things that can go wrong was very daunting. Max was poorly Monday and Tuesday as they tried to take him off the Milrinone IV, but is coping very well now and is stable. Every time the phone rings, I think it might be a new heart! Paul has been to visit this weekend so that was good, but hard for Paul having to say goodbye. Max enjoyed Skype chats with his friend and with his cousins. He has built a Meccano red arrow. Harry has been staying with his best friend, Will, from primary school this weekend, so he will have enjoyed that. He is also getting used to using the school bus. Took Paul to The Victory Pub last night, but neither of us have great appetites at the moment, so we had a starter. Need to start thinking about work soon. Clown Doctors are coming tomorrow so Max is looking forward to that. All our love and thanks for registering for these updates. Love Em X

"Lovely to chat last night and hear that Max is settled again on his Milrinone. You and Paul are doing an amazing job and are such strong people, keeping positive in such difficult circumstances. Harry and Max are very lucky boys to have such great parents. Keep strong and positive, xxx Charlotte."

"Hi, Emma. That all sounds positive news about Max. It must be so hard for both yourself and Paul with being so far apart and having to say goodbye to Max after the weekend. I hope you receive the phone call soon that Max has been found a new heart, as I am sure this will be a huge relief. Who are the Clown Doctors? Do they come around the ward in big feet and a spinning bow tie? Please pass on all my love and best wishes to Max and tell him how much we are all thinking about him at St Oswald's. Love, Alex X."

"Hi, Max and all! Glad to hear you are keeping busy building Meccano. I think you will make a great engineer. However, a Royal Navy submarine would be far more interesting than an RAF jet! I will look out for one :-) Keep smiling pal, as I know you will! Love, Neil, Benni, Jonni and the chickens x."

"Hi, Max and Emma. Just a quick line tonight to say 'Hi'. I think it was clowns today. Max, if you have a dream about eating a giant marshmallow, don't do it. In the morning, the pillow will be gone. Why did the physics teacher break up with the biology teacher? There was no chemistry. Bye for now. Nic."

"Sending you so much love. Will pop in soon to see you all. Love Norma."

Even before Emma and Norma Foster became firm friends, they worked closely and on a professional level. Norma was always very helpful and warm towards Emma.

They dropped out of touch when their work together ended. We didn't know how long we would be in Newcastle waiting for that gift of life, but Emma recalled that Norma lived nearby and that it might be nice to see a friendly face and hook up for a drink. Emma reached out to Norma and they duly arranged to meet at 'The Victory Pub'. From that night, their friendship grew. She loved our little Max and he adored her too. Norma had a wonderful way with children and with people in general; she became part of our family whilst we were living in Newcastle. She would visit Max, usually in possession of watermelon for Max and cake for us. She was so loving and supportive, even visiting Max when Emma and I were travelling to and from Newcastle. I have no doubt that we would have struggled a lot more than we did if we hadn't had Norma in our new Geordie lives.

Emma's friendship with Norma helped to take her mind off the precarious situation that Max was in. She also got to know me and Harry, who always seemed to be able to open up with Norma and express his bottled-up feelings about what was happening. Norma always made Emma feel that we were doing the right thing raising awareness about organ donation. Emma truly appreciated that Norma had a lovely spiritual circle who were championing Max's need for a heart and willing him to get the call that he so desperately needed.

DIARY OF A HEART MUM: Second Weekly Update – Sunday, 29 January 2017.

A difficult start to the week as Max had tummy pains and was very peaky, tired and fragile. By Tuesday, the decision was made to increase his Milrinone from 0.5 to 0.7. This is the maximum he can go to. Since the dose was changed, he is perky and stable with only occasional tummy pains. If he can be sustained on the new dose of Milrinone until the new heart arrives, we will be happy! However, today (Sunday) was a bad day, with Max struggling with his breathing, tummy ache and vomiting. The drugs will be assessed. Too poorly to dress, Skype or play today. Two steps forward. One step back! He did perk up a bit later in the afternoon though, so that was good! When he has been feeling well, Max has been kept busy with craft and games and he is enjoying his school session with Helen every day. He made a volcano and is busy making planets out of balloons to decorate his area. (Thanks to Norma for the idea and the earth and stars!)

Mum, Dad and Marcus visited from Monday–Wednesday, which Max enjoyed. Had a lovely meal at their hotel – Thanks, Mum and Dad! We discovered an amazing authentic Italian restaurant, which has an affordable 'happy hour' meal and is within walking distance of the hospital.

I went in to Newcastle on the Metro, vibrant city with beautiful architecture… Saw the film 'Passengers' – the message being to make the best of negative situations, which is what we are all trying to do! Also, was allowed free entry to the David Lloyd club around the corner from the hospital, so I could watch the indoor tennis, have a swim and sauna and eat a healthy meal!

Still enjoying The Victory Pub for an occasional hour of solace from 19–20. Delicious Mussels!

Went to Norma's house on Friday for dinner. It felt weird being in a proper house! Must be institutionalised, as I was hearing 'phantom beeping!' Ha ha! Thanks, Norma, the food and company was lovely! Nigel (Gramps) visited today, so that was nice for Max and he has delivered my car for me, so I now have wheels!

Max and I are learning the lingo here; try saying 'beta-blockers' in Geordie!

The lovely Harry and the lovely Paul arrived Friday night. So great to spend the weekend together as a family.

Finding people who can't contain their colds hygienically distinctly annoying, as I worry about Max catching a cold. Harry said, "Ignorance is the bane of humanity!" Ha ha!

Max said, "It's been an all right week and I'm feeling a little bit tired! I am looking forward to being given a new heart." Thank you for all the lovely cards and messages and sorry if I struggle to reply quickly.

"Hi, Emma and Max in Newcastle and Paul and Harry in Cheshire. So sorry to hear you've had a tough week – it must be pretty exhausting for all of you. However, on the plus side, it's great that you're all staying strong and positive, and that's really what helps to get things done and sorted. I'm going to an Angel workshop next Saturday and I'll be asking them all to continue watching over you and sending big love, light and healing to comfort and keep you all safe. Sending my own love, hugs and healing too. Stay strong. Maria"

"Hi, Emma and Max. Thank you so much for the update. It sounds like an up-and-down week with Max but lovely to hear you were able to spend a family weekend together with the lovely Paul and Harry (nothing beats family time). I have been telling the children at school recently that Max just had a 'poorly heart' but broke it to them all last week in assembly that he was going to need a transplant and explained what that meant. Pass on my love to Max. Warmest wishes to you all as always, Alex"

"Sending you all much love and hope you are having lots of fun with the clown doctors, who should be around today if I remember correctly. I can't wait to see the planets and volcano when I next come round to visit – awesome job, Max! Norma"

"Hi, Max. Just to prove to you I can master this bit of technology too (with your help, I have got the hang of the mobile phone as well now). Everyone at St Chad's is missing all of you – and looking forward to having you back with us. In the meantime, don't forget, its 'beta-blockers, pet'. Say hi to the gang. Love from Chris and all at church. XXXX"

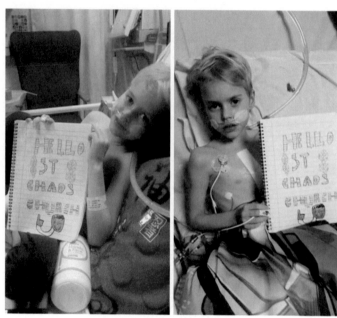

Max's message to St Chad's Church
Photo Credits: Emma Johnson

Chapter 4

It was the last weekend in January when Max hit one of those awful down draughts. Up until this point, he had been on Milrinone and he had worked his way up to the maximum permitted dose. On the Sunday, when the doctors did their ward round, it was clear he was struggling. By now, an increasingly familiar formation was coming together, spelling out the urgent need for further support. Not only was he complaining of a poorly tummy; a classic symptom of his heart failure, his breathing was shallow and rapid. More of a pant than a steady, deep rhythm. What was truly disconcerting, though, was the gallop his heart had developed. When the doctor placed the stethoscope on his chest, it bounced up and down, in time with the increasingly rapid beating of Max's heart. Something needed to be done.

I had to travel back to Cheshire with Harry, so that he could return to school. He'd spent the week with us after the news of Max's need for a transplant had been confirmed. I had been due to take Harry to stay with a friend, but he had wept uncontrollably in the car – the poor little boy – this was tearing him apart and he needed to spend some time with his brother. We got back to Cheshire and spent a fitful couple of days just existing when, mid-evening on the Wednesday, the phone rang and it was Emma. The team had been discussing Max at their meeting and it was decided that he needed to be fitted with a Left Ventricular Assist Device (LVAD). Our transplant consultant had mentioned the possibility of this being required when we'd had our discussion, but the shock was still palpable.

Max was to be operated on the following day, so I dropped a slightly more settled Harry with our friends and made the trip up to Newcastle, arriving just after midnight. The next day, we were met by the LVAD coordinator, Andrew, who showed us a 'demonstrator' of the device that was to be placed inside Max's heart and sealed in his chest, save for a wire which would exit Max's abdomen and provide power and instruction to the pump. We were handed a surprisingly large and heavy – although exquisitely made – metal lump, which looked like a Babybel cheese with a cheesy Wotsit sticking out of one side, a bit like a chimney. Apologies for the cheesy (pun intended) and ever so slightly mixed metaphor, but I hope it gives you an idea of the shape. Then again, maybe not. This sample unit, made out of titanium with a solid gold impeller was left with us to examine at our leisure. We were then visited by the anaesthetist, and this spelled a return to the serious, lay it all bare honesty that has to underpin such conversations. We were signing the consent forms for the operation – we would be allowed into the theatre itself, until Max fell asleep. We were warned, however, that Max may have a cardiac arrest as the anaesthetic was administered, due to the parlous state of his heart. Should this happen, we would be escorted from the theatre, but we must be assured that they were prepared for such an eventuality. Goodness me.

Forms signed, we returned to Max and he sat on my lap in his theatre gown and we waited for the theatre trolley to collect him. When it arrived, my heart was thumping – the trolley had steep sides and a narrow trough into which Max would lie. By this time, the 'premeds' had started to take their effect, and Max was swinging manically from tears to laughter; we were told that he would not remember this, but I wondered if his emotional volatility was representative of the fear and apprehension he was feeling. Max took with him a small, cuddly monkey – a gift from our tennis club friends – which now had a surgical facemask on. Rather unimaginatively, he was hurriedly named 'Monkey', but may I proffer that it would be a tad unfair to expect much effort being expended into the naming process under our somewhat extenuating circumstances!

We put on our surgical gowns and accompanied Max into the operating theatre. One of the surgical team and the anaesthetist performed a little comic routine for Max as he was wheeled in – they were brilliant. My stomach performed a one hundred and eighty degree flip as I walked into the brightly lit theatre. Over in the corner, I could see a huge table, the contents of its surface hidden from view by multiple towels. Seeing the instruments underneath would not, I surmised, be a good idea. To the right was the machine, which would keep Max alive as the surgeons fitted the pump to his heart, and then around the walls and the operating table, were banks of monitors and drip pumps, and in the middle of all of this, lying on the heated air mattress, was our little boy. Not for the first or last time, he looked so delicate and vulnerable, like the proverbial rabbit caught in the headlights of a car. As he lay there, his hair soaked with sweat, we caressed his head and tried to calm him – speaking was almost impossible – our tears were desperate to be unleashed, but we wanted to hold ourselves together. Our son was about to have major, open-heart surgery and we had been told he had a twenty percent chance of not making it. As the anaesthetist administered the anaesthetic, we gently urged Max to have sweet dreams – he'd already requested a dream about the Power Rangers from the anaesthetist. As his eyes glazed, he said, "Why do I feel so sleepy?" and then he was gone. We leaned forward and kissed him…as I lifted my face away from his, I couldn't help it; I turned and burst into tears. I may just have had my last kiss with my son, seen him alive for the last time; the emotion was all-consuming. I had never felt anything like it before, my insides were being wrenched and it was suffocating. We made it outside where the play specialist was there to offer comfort to us, and in time, the tears stopped to be replaced with a tense, nervousness as we awaited the outcome of this first round of major surgery.

We went to The Victory Pub! We didn't drink any alcohol…I don't think… but we had a small bite to eat – we didn't feel like much, as you would perhaps expect. A knotted stomach is a great appetite suppressant. Both of our phones were on the table and we checked incessantly for a signal, and to ensure that we hadn't missed a call. Upon returning to Scott House early evening, we took up residence in the main lounge and waited for news. As we had done with the papers at Leighton, we now did with the evening's televisual offerings; pretended to be interested, but paid scant regard to them. At around 23:30, our resolve crumbled – Max had been gone for some seven and a half hours and we had heard nothing – so we called PICU. They informed us that the surgery was over and that Max was just being tidied up in theatre. He would be arriving on the ward soon. He'd made it. *Thank you.* Half an hour later, we were outside PICU, being asked to sit in the parents' waiting room – the nurse would be out to speak with us shortly. After what seemed like an eternity, a nurse in salmon pink scrubs came out and told us that Max was on the ward and that the surgeon would come and brief us presently. At the earliest opportunity, we would be allowed in to see Max.

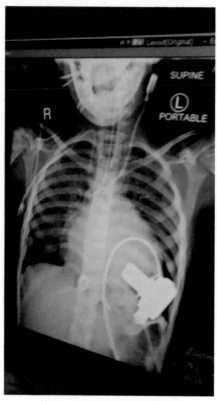

Max's X-ray showing LVAD
Photo Credit: Emma Johnson

When we eventually entered the ward, washed our hands and put on our plastic disposable aprons, we made our way to the second bed space along, which is where Max was now lying. It was a devastating sight. Max had tubes and drains coming from all over his little body, and there was a long, white rectangular plaster running from the top of his chest to just under his sternum. A breathing tube entered the right corner of his mouth with an unnerving sticking plaster mask holding the tube in place. He had probes on his head and a spaghetti-like array of tubes and wires making their way to the stacks of machines located behind his bed. In the corner was his main vital signs monitor, showing figures and squiggly lines, with which I was to become all too familiar. At the bottom of his bed, on a table, was a laptop, a plastic box, power transformers and batteries. This was the HeartWare Left Ventricular Assist Device control system and associated power supply. I could see numbers on the laptop screen; 1.8 this, and 1400 that and a squiggly line, perhaps showing the drive phase, but I wasn't sure. Max's eyes were slightly open, but unseeing; it was disconcerting. What did strike us most starkly was that he was wearing a nappy. The poor little boy had regressed – another one of those metaphors for his vulnerability and utter dependency on others for his very existence.

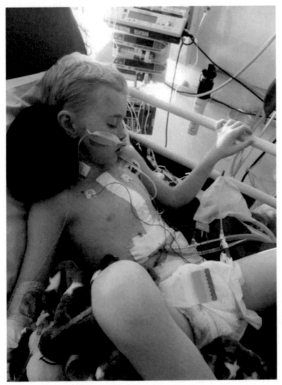

Max after having LVAD fitted
Photo Credit: Emma Johnson

We returned to Scott House completely exhausted; port after stormy seas. I looked at the phone in the corner of the room on the bedside cabinet and prayed that it wouldn't ring to summon us back to the ward. Mercifully, it didn't. The next morning, we made our way back to PICU, and whilst Max was still falling in and out of consciousness, he was starting to come 'round.

It was at this point that something happened, which shook me to my core and had a lasting impact on my psychological resilience and wellbeing. As I stood by his bedside, I looked at the monitors in the corner behind him. The numbers tumbled then rallied, up and down like a small boat being unrelentingly tossed on a stormy ocean. As I regarded this restless sea of uncertainty, the values on one line started to drop; slowly at first, but gathering momentum, like a runaway train. I glanced over at Max's nurse and he initially hadn't noticed. However, as I looked at him, silently yelling for him to see what I was seeing, I registered the obvious ignition of the mental processes which confirmed that he had locked onto this developing drama. His face maintained the smile it had on it before, as though his brain were too distracted to change it, but his eyes betrayed a growing sense of concern. He called over to the sister. The numbers were now in freefall – it was Max's blood pressure. Alarms started to sound and in a thrice, nurses were surrounding his bed. They spoke with Max, but by this time, the lack of blood – any blood – to his brain had caused him to crash. He was unresponsive. I found myself being moved further and further back, until I was almost against the corridor wall. Max's blood pressure was 21 over 19; a figure that will stay with me forever. Floating in a dizzying state of shock at the end of Max's bed, I honestly thought to myself, *this is it…I'm witnessing my son die*. I felt physically sick, pulled down by the weight of gravity and feeling increasingly desperate…*come on…do something*. I had witnessed this crisis unfold from its genesis and this is how it was all going to end, right here and now. I found myself willing Max on. *Do not go gentle into that good night, rage, rage against the dying of the light.* Working quickly as a team with instinct, experience, training and their finely tuned wits – everything which qualifies you to be working at this sharpest end of medical practice – the staff opened one of Max's necklines and injected huge quantities of liquid. Thankfully, this pulled things back from the brink as quickly as we had so frighteningly lunged towards it. The PICU consultant, who was now standing next to me, said, "It (the LVAD) is a mechanical device, it can go wrong." Yet again, a pummelling reality unleashed on us, but inescapably true – maybe it had malfunctioned. Fortunately, the LVAD was working okay. However, the experience, the rapidity with which it unfolded and the speed with which it concluded – and how in my mind it could so easily have ended – left a lasting, damaging impression on me. It caused a psychological scar that took away some of my resolve and ability to cope. How on earth would we get through this perfect storm?

Max's need for his first feeding tube was clear by the last week in January. Talk about helping Max to gain weight with a feeding tube (Naso-Gastric Tube or NGT) had finally come to a denouement and it was decided that he would have the tube placed through his nose and into his tummy the following day. Whilst Emma was nervous about this, she had no idea quite how traumatic this relatively straightforward (or so she thought) procedure would be.

Everything was ready and Max was even resigned to this decision, but nothing prepared Emma for his reaction. Two nurses worked as a team to put the tube down Max's nose. Emma could tell he was starting to get panicky as the tube went down. Once it was in, he went ballistic and screamed and screamed for the nurses to "Get it out!" He was hysterical and incandescent with rage for one and a half hours, screeching and crying. Emma felt so helpless, especially when Max cried out, "Mum, I'm choking!" She had never felt so afraid for her son and so helpless at the same time. She sat behind him on his bed and held him, trying in vain to calm him down. Max's heart-wrenching pleas for help were starting to have an effect on other parents, who in dribs and drabs, left the ward, as it must have been so difficult for them to hear Max's distress. Emma had to muster every ounce of strength not to burst into tears, but she had to stay calm to try and soothe Max. Nothing worked. The nurses were starting to get concerned, so they called for an X-ray technician, who could double-check that the tube was in the right place. Fortunately, the X-ray lady was able to reassure Max that the tube was correctly placed, and somehow, miraculously, managed to calm him down.

It took a few days for Max to recover from this ordeal. He would sit motionless staring out of the window at the 'Tree of Life' and Emma became increasingly concerned about his psychological well-being. It felt to Emma as if he had lost a piece of his soul, as his eyes were glazed over and his spark was snuffed out. After a few days, with the help of the psychologists, nursing staff and play specialists, he started to recover his spirit, and whilst uncomfortable, he seemed to be getting used to the tube. The decision to fit the LVAD removed some of the attention from the tube, which remained in place for a week or two after the LVAD operation, but was then removed and the dreaded regime with the apple 'juice' was started.

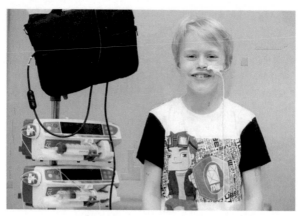

Max with LVAD machinery and IV medication
Photo Credit: Andy Commins/Mirror Newspaper Group

DIARY OF A HEART MUM: Third Weekly Update – Sunday, 5 February 2017.

What a week! We had a terrible time on Tuesday whilst Max had a feeding tube put through his nose. He genuinely thought he was choking. The crying and anguish went on for 1.5 hours. Luckily, the X-ray lady managed to calm him down. I think everyone on the ward was traumatised and I just felt completely helpless!

On Wednesday, the doctors and cardiologists had a meeting and decided that the left side of his heart was too precarious to risk leaving him with just Milrinone IV. So, the decision was made to fit a 'HeartWare' left ventricular assist device (LVAD). This was fitted in a 7.5-hour op on Thursday. He was accompanied by his monkey that Winsford Tennis Club bought him. The surgeons were amazing, but it was strange watching him fall asleep. He held his own mask and then said, "Why do I feel so sleepy?" The night before the op, met up with an old friend from Sale and Altrincham musical theatre who now lives in Gateshead at The Victory Pub. Took my mind off the next day.

Also, managed to meet up with Charlotte and Paul, who were celebrating their 10ᵗʰ wedding anniversary and were staying nearby. We went to The Victory Pub for lunch. Thank you, Lottie and Paul for treating us and for the cool hydraulic arm which Max will love when he starts to recover. We managed to have a giggle despite the circumstances.

Max had a couple of low blood pressure moments on Friday, which scared us a bit. He was away with the fairies, so wouldn't know anything about it. Still compos mentis enough to manage to find the remote control to adjust his bed and to try and peel off the plaster around his mouth! On Saturday, they stopped the ventilation and Max was breathing for himself. Still zonked out with Morphine and some sedative. Slight raised temperature, so they are watching for infection. Also, the right side of Max's heart is being supported by Milrinone, as the function is slightly impaired due to all the trauma.

Yesterday (Saturday) afternoon, Max's breathing tube was removed and he was breathing for himself. I got a cuddle with him whilst they changed mattresses, which was lovely, but I was worried sick about disturbing an important tube or wire! He is a lot more comfortable now. He is sleeping a lot due to drugs and when he does wake briefly, he is not happy at all about all the tubes and the nurses have to watch him like a hawk, as he may try and pull important tubes out. His temperature went back to normal today, so fingers crossed.

Paul and I felt exhausted on Saturday and spent our day either seeing Max or napping in our room at Scott House which is funded by the wonderful Sick Children's Trust. We are so blessed to have this facility to use as a home from home during our stay in Newcastle. Today, Max is a little more awake, but still away with the fairies. Paul is going home today to look after Harry and sort things out at home. Thank you all again for the amazing kindness and support. Love, Emma XXXX

"Emma – we are all glad to hear that the operation went well and that Max has since shown a sign of steady improvement. He is a tough little man and such a credit to you, Paul and his big bro! It sounds like Max is in very capable hands and it is reassuring that you have fantastic support locally from all the differing organisations (Pub Included) – The Chapmans"

"Hi, Em…It's so good of you to take time out to give us all such an in-depth update on Max. Makes it all so real and certainly helps me to try and imagine what you're going through. Positive thinking and prayers are very powerful – especially when they come in the quantities coming your way – so, hopefully, this will help you to stay strong and focus sometimes on looking ahead to the time when Max *is back home and free of all medical tubing! Bless him – he's such a trooper, isn't he? Really pleased you've managed a bit of social activity and guess it's much needed to recharge your own batteries. So good to have met up with friends whilst away from home too. See, you are being watched over and looked after from above as well as down here. Sending much love and hugs, Maria xxxx"*

"Thanks for keeping us all up to date. We are continuing to pray for him at St Peter's. Looking forward to seeing you when Max is ok for visitors again. Think The Victory Pub is a real godsend and can't wait to sample it! Love, Anne"

"Hello, Emma, really pleased to hear Max got through his op with no complications after the problems with feeding tube. You must have been made up to get that cuddle! I'm sure he will be more himself once the drugs are out of his system. It's an awful situation you are going through but I'm really pleased to hear that you and Paul met up with your friends and had some quality time together. I hope it made you feel a little more normal, albeit if it was only for a short time. I hope Max continues to improve now his LVAD has been fitted. Looks amazing, by the way, it's so inspiring seeing what these wonderful, clever, dedicated surgeons can do. I lit a candle for Max at Mass last night. We send our love and prayers to you all and we are thinking of you. Big hugs xxxx, Liz F"

It took Max a few days to adjust to life with an LVAD. For a while he was lost in the mental haze caused by the powerful cocktail of drugs he was on. On occasion, he would hallucinate – Max was convinced that there were babies behind him trying to pull him off the bed – the reality was that this pulling was caused by that spaghetti mess of tubes and wires. He also feared scary faces on the TV screen even though the TV was off. It is not easy seeing one so young and vulnerable so terribly distressed by the tricks his mind was playing on him. Our consolation was twofold; the effects of these drugs would be temporary and hopefully, the operation had stopped his glider from slamming into the ground. As the effects of the drugs wore off, Max was somewhat withdrawn and at times one sensed anger from him towards us. I think it was at this point that Max truly realised for himself, just how serious the situation was.

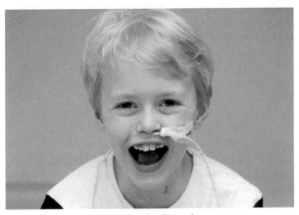

Max with feeding tube
Photo Credit: Andy Commins/Mirror Newspaper Group

DIARY OF A HEART MUM: Fourth Weekly Update –
Sunday, 12 February 2017.

Max had a really tough time post-op and has struggled to get back to his normal self. He couldn't stand the oxygen tubes in his nose and the feeding tube feels like a hair down your throat, so he hasn't wanted to swallow. On Wednesday, Max's physical progress was good enough that the necklines and drain lines from his heart were removed.

By Thursday, the oxygen tubes and feeding tube were removed. He can and must now eat, as the prospect of putting the feeding tube back is never far away! Max's mood lightened and he started to feel like his normal self. He has been telling me about weird memories of when he was away with the fairies. He thought that a scary baby was sitting behind him pulling on him and he could see three scary faces on the TV screen. He said that he felt really angry, but that he is OK now. He also said that he had a dream about a little boy who was sad and staring up into the sky, but that little boy has gone now. I asked if that little boy was Max and he said yes and that the real Max has come back! The psychologist, Kathryn, had a good chat with him on Tuesday, so that helped. She has given me some relaxation worksheets to do with Max e.g. The Treehouse, The Hot Air Balloon etc., and they really work well. He had some strange leg twitches (The neurologists ruled out seizure) and a bad trembling reaction to a temperature, but other than that, he is going from strength to strength. The physiotherapists are trying to build Max's strength, but he is very weak and gets tired easily. He was cheeky this morning, as the play specialists asked if he wanted to play a game and he said, "Yes, let's play the 'How long can I sleep' game," as he was desperate to be left alone to rest. Not surprising as it's still only just over a week since the op.

Max was measured for a wheelchair on Friday morning, which will be organised by our local authority. The hope is that if he can be weaned off the Milrinone for the right side of the heart, that he could go home, until the call for a new heart comes. They will design a special body vest that he can wear and which will hold Max's battery pack and machine. He may tire though as it is heavy, so will need the wheelchair.

Clair, the specialist cardiac nurse from Manchester, came to visit Max on Friday, so that was lovely for us. The Victory Pub is still keeping me sane.

Thank you for the beautiful cards that have been sent to the hospital. Max has loved getting his bundles of mail and we love looking at the cards together. They have pride of place on the wall.

"Thank you Max and Emma for the great news. Max has turned a corner and it looks like the road ahead is less bumpy for you all. All the positive things that are happening around you show a good and happy pathway ahead. Love to Harry and Paul and to you Emma and the incredibly brave and courageous Max! Malcolm and Sue x"

"Thanks so much for the update, Em. Max has had such a tough time (and all of you of course) but he sounds as if he is now back to being Max – an adorable, fun loving boy. He is amazing and in the midst of your worry, you must be very proud of your two boys for the way they've coped with this! Have a good week together! Maybe a small wine from time to time, Em? Much love from us all xxxxx, Janis"

"Thanks for the update, Emma. That sounds so much more positive after a tough week; it must be so wonderful to be talking about him possibly going home soon! Keep strong all of you. Loads of love as always. Love, Clare xx"

"That's positive, Emma, and good news. Thank you for taking the time to draft such a detailed summary. Much appreciated. Gosh, what a rollercoaster! You're all doing so well – whether it feels like

it or not – you are! We're all here for you. As always, love and light to you all xxxx, Suzanne"

After about a week, Max was moved back downstairs into the High Dependency Unit, with HeartWare LVAD computers, batteries and power supplies all stacked at the end of his bed for the short journey. For a time after his operation, Max had been pushing a raised temperature, and it was thought that there might be an infection at work. As a consequence, he was placed onto antibiotics. Our good friends and neighbours, Neil and Jonny, came to visit Max one Sunday, and we had a lovely day with them. We were in Newcastle as a family, so the three of us had settled down for the night in our room in Scott House, having said goodnight to Max. It was at around 11.30 p.m. when the phone in the corner of the room screeched into life. It was the ward. Max had taken a turn just as he was being given his medication – could we come over immediately. Emma was out of bed and dressed hurriedly, we didn't say much; we didn't need to. In the blink of an eye, Emma necessarily rushed on ahead and I was left in the room with Harry. The phone rang again. This time, it was the doctor speaking, checking that we were en route. "Should I come?" I heard myself asking. What a ridiculous question…of course I should. Again, it was the fear I felt rising inside me and my doubts regarding my ability to cope. That bloody scar. I felt angry with myself and I would subject myself to much opprobrium during the months of Max's illness for many reasons, but this stomach-churning fear and panic about facing the situation was by far and away my biggest frustration with myself.

I left for the ward, leaving Harry locked in the room. Perhaps not what I should have done, but I had no idea what was waiting for us and I didn't want Harry walking blindly into a situation like this. Whatever the outcome, I determined that it needed to be handled with consideration and control where Harry was concerned. I walked down the Magnolia Mile, my feet somehow disconnected from my consciousness, my mind racing and exploding with all sorts of devastating possibilities. It is hard not to fear the worst at such times, even though one should wait for the facts to be confirmed; then unleash the appropriate emotion. If only it were that simple.

As I rounded the corner at the end of The Mile, one of the nurses from the ward, Maria, stopped me. Max was being taken up to the intensive care unit. He'd had a reaction to one of the medications, but they were unsure, due to his condition, whether it had done any lasting damage to his brain. Maria did not want me coming across Max as he was wheeled out of the ward and taken upstairs. Typically thoughtful of Maria and appreciated. As she spoke, Max's bed appeared from the ward and entered the lobby and into the lift. I was ushered onto the ward and joined Emma, who had been shown through to the rest room. We were quickly escorted upstairs and seated in the long, thin parents' waiting room belonging to the intensive care unit. Not for the first time we sat and looked at one another, the tears in our eyes all that needed to be seen to appreciate how we were feeling.

A nurse came out and told us we could go and see Max. He had been taken to a side area of the unit, where the three beds shared the space with presently unused items of machinery; ventilators, heaters, coolers, ECHO machines and, perhaps the most daunting one of the lot – the ECMO machine. Max was lying on his bed, crying and saying, "I don't want them, they hurt." He was talking about the oxygen probes, which were about to be inserted into his nostrils and which he'd had to endure after his operation. There he lay, nine years old and perhaps twenty kilograms wet through. He was out from under his sheet in just his underpants, his little body already battered and scarred. His hair was wet and his eyes were wide and filled with tears. It's only after the event and upon reflection that you truly assimilate the crushing hurt an image like that engenders in every fibre of your being. At the time, you want to soothe and take that pain away. Immediately, however, amidst this heartrending scene, there was a positive; the damage to Max's brain that had been feared had clearly not happened. He may have been small and utterly defenceless, but he was letting the team know in no uncertain terms that he did not want the nasal probes anywhere near him! The same consultant who only a few days earlier had said, "It's a machine – they do go wrong," stood by Max's bed. "He doesn't have to have the probes if he doesn't want them." Sound judgement, professional discretion, compassion – all in a breath. Instead, a small mask was produced, to give Max's battered little body the oxygen it craved and it did the trick; Max settled and soon dropped off to sleep. We left for the ward to collect Harry, who had been fetched from Scott House by two of the nurses; I was glad – it was a good call. Fortunately, the conversation with him was not going to be the difficult, devastating one we had at first feared.

When you are in this sort of situation, with a gravely ill child, your thoughts primarily centre on your predicament, but the plight of others is not lost on you. Oh no. When Max had this anaphylactic shock, caused by one of his antibiotics, several parents were on the ward with their babies. The following morning, I spoke with one of the fathers, who recounted the experience. As Max started falling, the doctor administering his medication raised the alarm. Now, one gets used to buzzers and alarms on the ward – they are pinging and shrieking all of the time. This alarm, however, was described as something completely different; an alarm to send a chill to the very core of the soul. Within only seconds, Max was surrounded by doctors from across the hospital, working frantically to bring him back. As this was being done, the parents were lead out of the ward and into the kitchen area; shocked and with a shattering appreciation of what they had witnessed. As he told me this, his eyes filled with tears – yes, you think of your own child and overlay the circumstances before you as though relating to them – in part, it's how we empathise. But it was more than that. Max was a little boy who could talk with people, laugh with them and build relationships with them. Parents on the ward could see his character, see him for the lovely little boy he was and they could see his suffering. You do bond with the other parents and children – heck, you are sharing something which profoundly affects all of you, and it is unquestionably experienced in adversity. So, the tears were from the heart; to hear of the death of a child on the ward is devastating, but to be there when it happened…

It is an inescapable, inevitability of life in a department caring for children with chronic heart problems; death is always lurking. Despite the best, all out efforts of the medical team, there are children who came onto the ward during our stay, who did not make it. It is all part of the contradictory, diametrically opposed emotions you feel about your situation.

I will never forget early one morning as Harry and I were taking a break in Scott House, Emma returned to the room, crying inconsolably. Once she had calmed down sufficiently, she explained that she had been walking past the CHUF shop, when she came across one of the familiar 'heart mums' crouching against the wall in the corridor, a guttural cry from the mother cutting into Emma with such force, it is a sound she will never forget. Emma approached her, bent down and tenderly put an arm around her shoulder.

"Has something happened?" Emma quietly asked.

"She's gone!" the mother replied.

They both stood up and Emma held her, not quite knowing what to do next. "Oh, I'm so sorry!" she found herself saying. Quickly rounding the corner, a member of the nursing team appeared and promptly took over, gently leading this grief-stricken mother to a side room. For the rest of her life, Emma will remember this awful moment and thinks often of this family and the daughter they had just lost.

Chapter 5

The following morning, Max was taken back down to HDU. Emblazoned across his notes was the name of the antibiotic which, rather than make him better, had so nearly taken him from us. Also, a change of bed space – number four. I have always believed that nursing must be a vocation – a calling – to make a difference to the lives of people who are suffering, as well as their families. Many of the children on Ward 23 were babes in arms, but with Max, you had a little boy whose personality was already hard-wired. Over the months, one would see little things that the nurses did to keep him entertained and to make his time just that little bit more comfortable and in keeping with the nine-year-old boy he had just become.

As I've already alluded, getting a child with end stage heart failure to eat is not easy. It's not helped by the fact that his condition severely limited his ability to get out and about. Every day, we would endeavour to push the boundaries of his physical activity, to try and build him up and give his poor, ailing heart some exercise to keep what little function it had from taking leave of absence. It is very hard to see a previously fit and active little boy struggle to walk the short distance from his bed to the door of the High Dependency Unit – a distance of maybe twenty feet. Building him up was going to be a long, hard road but it is a road we simply had to travel. We searched for anything Max might eat, to keep his weight up. To add to his frustrations, he was severely restricted in the amount of fluid he was allowed to drink. One night, he was particularly thirsty and dry, so one of the nurses, Katie, went to have a look in the ward kitchen. In there, she found some ice pops in the freezer and gave one to Max. The satiating impact on his thirst, relative to the small volume was huge, and Max became dependent for a time on these frozen little miracles to keep him comfortable. Unfortunately, supplies were running low on the ward, so having had a few hours' sleep after her night shift, Katie made a special trip to the supermarket to buy further supplies – at her own expense – and brought them in for Max the following evening. McDonald's fries were another popular gastronomic gift giver for Max.

A nurse with whom he shared a close bond, Sophie, made a seven-mile round trip to the local McDonald's after a twelve-hour day shift, just to collect some fries for Max, who devoured them appreciatively. I would like to make mention a few more kindnesses. Whilst you may think hospitals are very clean, infection-free places, there are certain bugs which inevitably can and do wreak havoc on wards from time to time. Sadly, for Max, he picked up a couple during his stay. Norovirus is a most unpleasant illness, and a bout which hit Max resulted in him being placed in quarantine – literally confined to bed with 'Do Not Cross' tape alerting people to the hazard within; the Freeman's very own 'Chernobyl Elephant's Foot'. One of the nurses, Rachel, with whom Max had enjoyed much playful banter, extended his territory to the adjacent, empty bed space, and promptly procured most of the ward's spare sheets, so that she could make him a den. Max loved it. Other nurses were equally kind.

If it wasn't willingly taking Max for little walks around the hospital – and beyond – it was bringing their pet dog to the park opposite the hospital, so that Max could be introduced on a walk – Max loves animals. It wasn't just the nurses who consistently demonstrated these nameless acts of kindness and love, so typical of our experience.

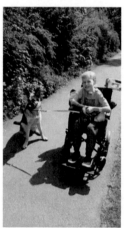

Max with German Shepherd, Sydney
Photo Credit: Paul Johnson

When you live – in effect, it was our second home – in such an intense environment for any period of time, you really notice the small things. One of the cardiologists, Stavros – a man of few words, but kind and gentle – would stroke Max's head after he had finished his examination and conclude with a high five.

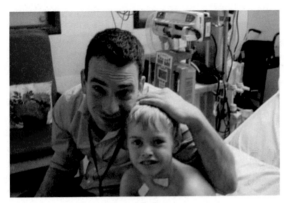

Max with Stavros
Photo Credit: Emma Johnson

Another, Andreas, brought in collectable football cards he had been saving for Max, who by now had developed quite a collection. Indeed, cards came in from all quarters, as staff across the department heard of Max's record-breaking array.

One's relationship with the staff is very personal to the individual, and to me it was extremely important. Half of my life was being played out in the hospital, so the doctors, nurses – the entire team – become an extension of one's family. As you have done for the entire life of your child, they too are now also responsible for his care, so the bond created can be very powerful. I found myself wondering how difficult it must be to maintain a professional distance, whilst ensuring that the emotional needs of both children and parents are acknowledged and addressed. I pondered how easy it would be to become close to a patient or their parents, and yet the need for self-preservation in this emotionally-charged environment is paramount. As I have poignantly referenced, not all of the children make it, therefore, the need to be engaging and compassionate – with a realistic degree of closeness – is quite a balance to achieve. Over friendliness could be so damaging emotionally. This team of people charged with doing all they could for our son, may yet have to sit us down and give us devastating news – how much harder this would be if the professional and emotional boundaries had become blurred. And yet, I needed their acknowledgement – even if it were just a nod in the corridor, it somehow validated me as a part of this broad family.

Many are the sayings and phrases which can be utilised to describe life as the parent of a gravely ill child. Life is full of ups and downs, bumps in the road, you take two steps forward and one step back and so you go on. It's a language you share with all of the other parents, who are also trying to deal with their own personal sadness, whilst continuing to function, however limited that function may be.

One of the most sustained dips in Max's condition came in the February, not long after his terrible reaction to the antibiotic. We had been visited by Max's Uncle Roger, Auntie Lucy and their three children, James, Edward and William. A portent of things to come had been Max's distance, his quiet yet distressing inability to engage with his brother and cousins. A trip to the playroom and a go on the FIFA 2015 computer game would normally see a relative spike in excitement, accompanied by occasional outbursts of frustration at a missed tackle or, worse still, a squandered chance in front of goal. On this occasion, there were no bug scuttling shots on target, instead Max sat quietly in his wheelchair and, after only one condensed half of Stoke versus Inter Milan, he asked to go back to his bed.

As we all sat around his space, he tried to rally, glimpses of his normal perky, cheeky little self, coming to the fore, but as his Auntie and cousins went for a walk in the adjacent Freeman Park with Emma, Max lay silent on his bed. Not for the first – or last – time during his stay in Newcastle, I became aware of a doctor standing by his charts, wearing green surgical scrubs. Max's medically wrought melancholy had been picked up during the ward round earlier in the day and his nurse had also observed him with a growing sense of concern. Now, the green-clad doctor spoke with the ward doctor and then quietly introduced himself as the intensive care unit registrar.

It is a fact of life on the heart ward, that children can yoyo between the ward and intensive care, as the fragility of their condition dictates and now it was Max's turn to be under the spotlight. The doctor spoke with me, and stated that Max's heart appeared to be struggling with the LVAD – in particular the right side of his heart – which was simply being overwhelmed. He told me that he had been asked to take a look at Max and plainly stated that it was likely he would need to be taken to intensive care, quite probably by the end of the day. In a bizarre, gallows-style reflex of humour, we had a bet that this would be the case. Only in times of such stress and only in order to cope, would you entertain such dark humour. Emma too found herself almost seeking humour to try and lighten the load: Nurse to Emma: "The doctors feel that it would be nice for Max to have a duvet."

Emma to nurse: "Du vet?"

Nurse to Emma: "Mmm…one side is bigger than the other…"

Emma to nurse: "Mmm…like Hitler's balls!" – it seemed the usual social filter just wasn't working!

When Max's Mum, cousins and Auntie returned to the ward, they said their goodbyes – Emma was heading back to Cheshire to look after Harry, but I could see the angst etched into every contour of her face; she could see that Max was fading. As they left, Max tried his best to be upbeat, but his condition simply repressed his natural desire to be engaging and funny; instead, he quietly thanked his extended family for visiting and gave his Mum a kiss. By now, dusk was announcing the end of the day and night was ready to assume its position of primacy. Normally, I would have read a story to Max and started to settle him ahead of the important business of sleep. However, tonight, he had already started to sleep. His advanced heart failure meant that lying flat on the bed caused him to become breathless, so he was propped up at a sixty-degree angle. In the now semi-darkness of the ward, I looked at him – he just didn't seem right. I took hold of his duvet, and moved it to one side. His breathing set off alarm bells immediately. I have a guilty confession – I have watched the YouTube video of Tommy Cooper's death on stage – I'm not proud of this voyeuristic act, but having read his biography, the inevitable internet search ensued. Why would I mention this? Quite simply, Max's breathing now reminded me of the dying, gasping convulsions in Tommy Cooper's body as he slumped to the floor and his eternal sleep.

I glanced to the left at the monitor hanging from the gantry over Max's bed and could see his heart was beating at 155 beats per minute – way too fast, even for Max. I called the nurse over; I didn't need to explain anything to her. In an instant, she sent for the doctor and I was gently pointed in the direction of the parents' rest room at the end of the ward. Immediately, I thought of my 'bet' earlier in the day – I knew in my heart of hearts that Max would be heading upstairs. Some half an hour had elapsed when Max's nurse came to fetch me and confirmed that he would be going to PICU. In the time that I had been gone, Max had been given some diuretics and had already peed out the perfect pint; he had been drowning in fluid, which his broken heart and body simply could not process. He

71

appeared more settled than before, but was distressed by the news that he was being moved upstairs to the intensive care unit; could you blame him?

We got Max settled in a side section of PICU and I then began the process of clearing his bed space in the High Dependency Unit. This is a right royal pain and, at the time, one feels aggrieved at having to do this onerous task, emptying drawers of clothes and books, electronic devices, loose felt tips and the like. However, upon reflection, it is largely stuff we'd brought into the hospital, so fair's fair – it is for us to gather this accrued detritus together, plonk it onto the metal trolley provided specifically for such moves, and head for its new home.

Over the following days, doctors worked to stabilise Max and, again, a carefully considered concoction of drugs, including adrenaline, allied with a recalibration of his LVAD, steadied the ship to a degree. However, Max's lack of appetite meant that his weight, bearing in mind he was nine, had dropped to twenty kilos (roughly three stone). Food consumption was a constant battle, and the fitting of his first feeding tube had been a truly traumatic event for all concerned. To this day, Max still suffers flashbacks to the experience of getting the tube in place and the terrible distress it caused. Certain foodstuffs were acceptable to Max, but not to our bank balance; smoked salmon, strawberries and Jaffa Cakes were his staple diet. I also had to discipline myself not to eat all the Jaffa Cakes…I confess I had to replace quite a few packets.

When you live with the chronic stress caused by having a critically ill child, it takes its toll physically, mentally and spiritually. We were in a situation over which we exercised no control, we had no idea how long it would go on for and, perhaps most damaging of all, didn't know how it was going to end. One tries not to think 'worst case scenario', but on the occasions when Max hit a down draft, the fineness of his corporeal thread was starkly apparent; we could barely see it. Every so often, usually when Max was at a low ebb, I became aware of one of the surgeons standing nearby; at a sufficient distance from Max's bed to be out of the engagement orbit, but close enough to exert gravitational pull – you were only too aware of their presence.

You will not, I suspect, be surprised to learn that we had huge admiration and respect for the surgical team looking after Max. Mr Asif Hasan and Mr Fabrizio de Rita fitted Max's LVAD pump to his badly broken heart. Staff across the department spoke of Mr Hasan, the lead surgeon, and Fabrizio, with such respect – it was clear that they were revered and liked by everyone. When the surgeons visited the ward, we always wondered with a frisson of excitement if they were coming to prepare Max for his transplant. They would quietly enter the ward to see a patient and the team looking after them then, discussions over, they would depart without fanfare. Transplantation was one of their considerable skills. Other parents would recount acts of transformational brilliance carried out on broken hearts the size of a walnut. Such talented, humble men, fighting for every heartbeat and doing everything they can to turn hopes into reality.

When they visited Max in PICU, they would stand, arms folded across their chest, saying nothing, but the look on their largely enigmatic faces betrayed a sense of concern; Max needed to be well enough to receive his new heart. If his glider flew too low, then he would be off the transplant list and, barring a miracle, it would then only be a matter of time.

As a parent, you registered these visits, the looks, the comments between professionals. This, in part, is why the whole process was so draining; you were aware of everything and overdosing on adrenaline. There is much to be said here about not reacting to something that hasn't happened; we knew the team were completely honest and would share their concerns, but it is impossible not to be buffeted and hurt by what you see and hear, even if at times a little knowledge can be very dangerous.

We were lucky to have the support of two psychologists, Sue and Kathryn, who worked with Max and our family to help us develop ways of coping. For Max, some sense of routine and purpose was vital, as was giving him a means of expressing how he was feeling at any given time. As a result of his chats with Kathryn, his bed space became filled with charts and drawings, to help us all focus on keeping him motivated. I came to really appreciate my chats with Sue – something that I would never have considered prior to Max's illness. Sometimes, the meetings would take place outside, as the North East weather permitted. I would sit with her and talk of my fears for the here and now, and my fears for the future – the loss of a carefree life we had once known and the uncertainty and responsibility of the one with which we were now presented.

During these conversations, I faced up to the reality of losing my son; that he may not survive. I felt like I was in mourning. I was trying to prepare myself (although one can never be truly prepared for such heartbreak) for the worst case, which as Max lay in intensive care, seemed like a very real possibility. At night, I would dream of his funeral, seeing the faces of the mourners as we left the church behind his coffin. I would wake in the morning with tears on my cheeks and a leaden weight in my heart. I was mourning for the life we had lost, the stable existence we had so taken for granted. I was also mourning for Max, for the life he had lost. He always used to talk, with his childlike optimism and naivety, of living into his nineties; I cried for the reality of his future both in the short term and, if he were to be granted one, the long term. How I wished he had met my Mum, his amazing Gran, and how I yearned for her to be with me now. I have always felt the oppressive sadness of losing my Mum, but I now felt it with a greater pulling in my heart than ever. I would talk of how I struggled with certain elements of the day – that morning uncertainty – and why I sometimes had to walk around the outside of the hospital, rather than along Magnolia Mile, to reach Max. I wanted to take myself out of the shattering stress of the situation – I wanted it to go away, and a glimpse of sky and cars and the sound of birdsong in the park at the front of the hospital all granted me my fantasy, even if the 'Cardiothoracic Entrance' sign slammed me back into the as is. It was a conversation with another professional, away from the hospital, when it really hit home to Emma that we may very well lose our son. She was advised to try and undertake activities with Harry and me as a family of three, in case this was to become the norm. It was sound and very well-intentioned advice and in fairness, it would be impossible to make any such suggestion sound palatable. But it needed to be done. Somehow, we had to cover the bases and prepare as well as we could for the worst-case scenario. Believe me, every cell in our bodies was screaming for our little boy to make it, but the statistics are black and white – not everybody does.

Keeping Max motivated was going to be central to our efforts to bridge him to transplantation. Doctors worked miracles to prop up his badly broken heart, but at the nucleus of efforts to keep his spirits up were his family. Play specialists, psychologists and clown doctors added up to a magnificent support team, but the key people for Max were his Mum, Dad and brother. This was evident through his wish to have us with him, ideally at all times.

Emma, when she was on caring detail with Max, had a disciplined routine that she would stick to, and that allowed her the space to gather her thoughts and taste some semblance of normal life away from the hospital. Lunchtimes would see her power walk her way around Freeman Park to try and clear her head, whereas evenings saw her walk to The Victory for dinner, before returning to tuck Max into bed and head back to Scott House to watch Celebrity Britain's Big Talented Brother or other such televisual fodder. I, on the other hand, would seldom venture far from the hospital during the day, other than to stock up on smoked salmon, watermelon and to replace the Jaffa Cakes I'd scoffed. Evenings were equally limited in imagination. I would get Max ready for bed and just about have him settled for the 8 o'clock handover to the night shift. Occasionally, I would be expelled from the ward by the nurses; quite right, as they had to discuss the patients in turn and these discussions were not for public consumption. I would leave the ward, returning some thirty minutes later to get Max off to sleep, having overseen the administration of his night-time medications.

We would sit for a time, just chatting or watching a DVD and then Max would announce that his melatonin 'sleepy meds' had started to kick in and that he was ready to settle. This was my cue to dig out the latest book we were reading to him – he was a fan of David Walliams' *The Midnight Gang*, which is set in a children's hospital ward – and I would draw the curtains around his bed and start reading; I even tried to 'do' the voices for him.

As I read, Max would lie on his side and listen, as with my free hand, I did little swirly tickles on the palm of his hand. After a couple of chapters, I would look up, and almost without exception, would see that Max had fallen asleep. I joked with Max that I knew he was asleep, as the pillow was covered in sticky, translucent goo and he was snoring loudly. Although he fell for this first time – "Really?" he said – it only worked on the first occasion, but I persevered anyway. No, I actually knew he was asleep because his resting pulse rate dropped considerably. Sometime in July, it dropped below 100 beats per minute, which was the lowest I had seen it at any stage during his time in hospital. I would quietly stand up, put the 'big chair' back against the wall under the window next to the 'Tree of Life', blow him a little kiss and bid the nurses good night. "I'm on my mobile if you need me," I insisted on saying…yes, they probably thought, and you're on the end of an internal phone in Scott House, but we know what you mean. "Sleep tight," they would say.

Having returned back to my little den in Scott House for the night – anytime between 9:30 and 10:00 – I would complete my day of unwholesome, completely inappropriate food with a Pot Noodle, a bowl of Crunchy Nut Cornflakes and some After Eight Mints (on offer at the time!). In isolation, every so often, there is nothing wrong with these foodstuffs – just not almost every night. It's no wonder that Asda doesn't stock my clothing size! Mirth aside, there is a serious point. This whole thing was damaging our psychological wellbeing quite considerably – the need, therefore, to look after physical wellbeing was critical; Emma did a much better job of that than I.

To keep Max buoyed, we looked to try and give him something simple to focus on, to look forward to. At home, Max's bedroom was perhaps typical of the 'boy' breed. Full of clutter and half-completed projects, at the time he fell ill, his room was in much need of a revamp. His burgeoning collection of speakers and love of music and lights – he had a multi-coloured light ball, which illuminated his bed space and much of the ward at night – meant that he had a developing taste and knew what he liked. In part to keep me busy and mentally occupied whilst at home with Harry, I decided that I would redecorate Max's room. I told Max this, and his little eyes lit up and the tiny cogs in his brain started whirring. It's lovely to see that untainted look of excitement and gratitude in a child's eyes and Max relished the opportunity to shape the design of his 'new' room. This also provided a really useful tool to help keep him motivated.

"Whatever comes along to test us, Max, just think about your room, sitting in your big massaging chair listening to your music," I would say…you could see his mind picturing the scene and the whole idea gave him something to engage with and look forward to. What was heart-breaking for us was the issue of timing. At this stage, the reality was that he may never make it home to enjoy such a room, and whilst we lived with this gnawing, painful reality, the promise of a refurbished bedroom was unquestionably viewed as 'game on' by Max – it was going to happen. Believe me, nothing was going to give me greater pleasure than to give Max the best bedroom in the world, because to do so would mean that he was coming home in the manner we had prayed for.

DIARY OF A HEART MUM: Fifth Weekly Update – Sunday, 19 February 2017.

Max moved downstairs on Monday from intensive care to High Dependency Unit, as he was progressing so well.
He had a really good day on Tuesday, but on Wednesday morning, he seemed to deteriorate again, so they are trying to get his fluid balance right and have raised the Milrinone dose from 0.2 back up to 0.3 to support the right side of the heart. They are

also trying to get the right Heparin/Warfarin balance correct to get the blood the right consistency for the machine.

I took Harry into Newcastle City on the Metro on Tuesday and Wednesday. On Wednesday, we discovered the 'Catpawchino' cat café. It was brilliant and very relaxing. We walked over the Millennium Bridge on the River Tyne. Beautiful weather too!

Poor Paul is struggling and he wakes up very anxious every morning. However, he is enjoying building the robotic arm with Max which Charlotte and Paul bought. It is a big project, but Max loves it.

The doctor let me hear Max's heart through the stethoscope and it whirs like a machine! Well, I suppose it is a machine in there! We will soon have 'HeartWare' training so we know how everything works and what the different alarms are!

Max was introduced to another little boy, aged 10, who is due to have HeartWare fitted and the circumstances are very similar to Max. I have a feeling they will become hospital friends!

Thursday was good for most of the day. Our neighbours, Neil and Jonny, from across the road in Winsford came to visit and Max enjoyed Minecraft lego along with a very amusing joke book! We went to The Victory for tea. We managed to have a laugh and said our goodbyes. We settled back at Scott House for the night only to be called by the HDU ward, to say that Max was unwell. He had been started with some IV antibiotics due to an infection and poor Max had an allergic reaction (anaphylactic shock), which meant that his heart rate went right down, he went dizzy, couldn't see and then went unconscious and stopped breathing. He had a strange seizure too. Luckily, the nurses put out an emergency alert and everyone came running and rescued him. He was taken to intensive care and by the time we were able to see him, although distressed, he was definitely back to 'Max'!

By the end of Friday, he had bounced back and was taken back downstairs to the HDU ward! Panic over! They have worked out the particular ingredient that Max is allergic to and have now started a different IV antibiotic, which doesn't contain it!

We were all very drained by that experience, but we were very proud of Harry and how he coped so well! Max spoke to the psychologist about it, as we were worried he might have been frightened. He seemed OK and recounted what happened. He said that after feeling dizzy and not being able to see, he remembers being in a long cave with smooth walls and he was walking towards a bright light at the end of the cave. He then heard a whoosh noise and woke up! Very strange!

By Saturday, we were back on track with visitors again after having to cancel our Friday visitors. Uncle Roger, Auntie Lucy, James, Edward and William came to visit. We had lunch at The Victory, then came back to see Max. Max managed to walk to the playroom. Later on, Roger and Paul stayed with Max, whilst Lucy, me and the boys went for a river walk in the Freeman Park opposite the hospital. Dusted out the cobwebs. Thanks for the cookies, chocolate brownies, pictures and Amazon voucher. Very kind!

On Sunday, Nigel and Uncle Dan came to visit and as Harry and I said our goodbyes, Paul took them to The Victory for a light bite! Unfortunately, Max was very tired and the doctors explained that Max's liver had gone from 2 cm enlarged to 4 cm enlarged, which is a sign that the right side of the heart is struggling, so the Milrinone dose was increased to 0.4! His shoulder was really aching too. He really is a very frail little boy and it breaks my heart to see him suffering.

Harry and I dropped by at Mum and Dad's who took us to an Italian restaurant for some tea along with Uncle Marcus. Finally landed back at home Sunday evening. Home sweet home, but not the same without Paul and Max. A pile of post to plough through!

P.S: I would like to mention a remarkable little boy called Hugh, who has written a letter and four postcards to Max, as well as organising a choir recording of a song dedicated to Max, which he would like Max to listen to when he is feeling fragile. Hugh is such a thoughtful and kind little boy and Hugh's correspondence has really helped Max through this difficult journey. Thank you, Hugh!

"Hi Emma, you are becoming quite a medical expert with all the lingo! All the things Max, you, Paul and Harry have had to endure have been unbelievable. He is such a determined and resilient sole and I am sure this is what is helping him bounce back so many times from all the adversity. I wish you and Max a panic free week and hope that he continues to be on the mend in the HDU. All our love and best wishes to you all. Alex."

"Hi Em, thank you for the update but so sorry that it has been such a difficult time for Max and all of you. You must be totally drained. We're in awe of you all regarding the way you're all carrying on with such an incredible anxiety. Max is such a brave boy and it's great that he will have a new friend who is going through a similar time. They'll be able to support each other. Harry too is amazing and deserves huge hugs too! As always, you are all continually in our thoughts and we're willing Max on and back to good health. Much love, as always, from all the Finnigans xxx P.S: really would like to visit the 'Catpawchino' cat café!"

"Thanks for the update, Emma. Some good, some less so. Oh how I feel for you. Even at home, you can't relax. It's such an ordeal for everyone. Thank goodness, he is in such capable hands although it is so far away. I bet Max loves having Harry there, and another little boy in the same situation will be a great diversion, I feel sure. Thinking of you every day, and wondering how things are. You are brave and strong because you HAVE to be, but it's not easy and you must be exhausted emotionally xx, Liz C."

"What a rollercoaster week for you all and still you sound so positive in your posts. So pleased you're getting visitors. That must help. You're all never far from my thoughts. Just wish there was more I could do. Lots of love to you all and I pray for a less stressful week for you all. Love, Vicky. Xx."

Chapter 6

DIARY OF A HEART MUM: Sixth Weekly Update – Sunday, 26 February 2017.

Where to start! Last Sunday night, the docs were getting concerned about Max's breathing and function of the right side of the heart. His weight loss was also a concern. The decision was made to move Max back upstairs to PICU (Paediatric Intensive Care Unit) until stable. Max was given adrenaline and oxygen. Of course, Max was not very happy as he detests the tubes in the nose.

I had already arrived back in Winsford and found it impossible to go to work, so another false start. Will try again tomorrow! I enjoyed the little things I had missed – a Subway meal, a cappuccino at St Luke's coffee shop on Delamere Street, and I bought some great bargains at the British Heart Foundation charity shop! It was lovely to be back at Rose Cottage, but felt strange without Max and Paul. Harry was wonderful! P.S: He got a first-class school report, despite difficult circumstances.

On Tuesday night, Chris, the vicar of St Chad's and our church friends arranged to meet Harry and me at the Old Star Pub for drinks. Ernie, the landlord laid on a hotpot with red cabbage and bread! Thanks, Ernie. We managed to have fun and it did us good. Was very tired on Wednesday morning, though, as I set off for Newcastle. Arrived in Newcastle and when I saw Max, I could see the weight loss on his ribs and face. He looked so hollow eyed and the nurse told me he had dropped to three stone! They were seriously considering reinstating the feeding tube! However, they started a new feeding plan instead with some different high calorie drinks. On Thursday, he had gained weight and he did really well with his food and drink intake.

Thursday was also a terrible day for me, as I was told that Max's hospital friend had died. This really shook me and I was devastated. I still can't believe it… He was such a dear, sweet little boy. Max hasn't been told…yet! It drummed home to me the severity of Max's condition and the sadness that, had that little boy got a new heart in time, he would still be with his family. Truly awful! After consoling myself with a spritzer at The Victory, I returned to Max in PICU. Max was fast asleep, but instead of disappearing back to Scott House, I stayed until 22:00 watching 'Finding Dory' on DVD. After that news, I just needed to be near him!

On Friday evening, I met Norma at, you guessed it, The Victory Pub, and we really enjoyed the food. Thank you, Norma, for the 'global healing meditation' that you organised, just for Max. The messages that you showed to me were very moving! Also grateful to Norma, as she was given permission by the nurses to pop in today to sit with Max, as Sunday is the only day when occasionally Max doesn't have his Mum or Dad with him! She has made some very special, calorific watermelon flavour ice cream for Max!

On Saturday, Max's Godmother, Auntie Helen visited and we met for lunch at The Victory, and then I got permission for Helen to come in and see Max. Max was feeling a bit unwell, but soon perked up once he had been to the loo! He had been very constipated and it was making him breathless, with an overly high heart rate! They put Max's oxygen and adrenaline up! Thank you, Auntie Helen, for the cookies, watermelon etc. Thank you especially for organising the letter for Max from Manchester United, complete with Wayne Rooney signed card! Just wonderful!

It would appear that Max's heart needs the adrenaline. As long as he is on adrenaline, he will need to stay in intensive care. This means that he will be pretty much bedbound... The good news is that by today, Max's weight had increased to 22 kg! Thanks for all the lovely cards and letters. These really connect Max to the outside world! Love, Em X

"Hi, Emma, another mammoth week for you – words can't really put into context what you must be going through. It is really good news that Max is putting on weight and I am really not surprised you are not yet ready to return to work (I don't think anyone would be!). I am also pleased to hear Harry has got such a glowing report from his school – pass on my congrats to him! Love to you all, as always – Alex"

"Emma, you are amazing. As I've said I have no words but know we are thinking of you xx, Ben."

"This morning Gary and I went to church and the first thing we saw was a picture of Max with his message on the overhead projector. It was lovely and so good for folks to see as everyone asks after him regularly. We hope you have received or will soon receive Gary's postcard from his trip to Scotland which we all enjoyed. Sending love and prayers and a big smile from Gary as usual from Liz, Paul and Gary x"

"Hi, Emma, good news that Max has gained some weight. I bet his face lit up when he opened his card of Wayne Rooney, brilliant! So sorry to hear Max's hospital friend has died, that is just awful. Sending you lots of love and hugs, Em, and thinking of you all lots xx, Jac and Jeff xx."

"Max is definitely in the best of places to care for him so conscientiously. Max is an inspiration to us all when I read about the week's developments and how he is coping so incredibly well. Emma, you continue to be that special Mum, and with Harry and Paul to support you with all the love they can gather, we all hope and pray that Max will beat this. Love to you all every minute of every day. Malcolm xxx."

DIARY OF A HEART MUM: Seventh Weekly Update – Sunday, 5 March 2017.

A mixed week! Max had a wonderful afternoon last Sunday with Norma, who kept Max busy with colouring, games, watermelon and homemade ice cream.

I returned home on Sunday and tried to mentally prepare myself for work. Actually managed to go to work on Monday and Tuesday. The change of focus did me good. In a brand-new office with new furnishings and fancy bathroom and kitchen! Desk was ready and waiting. The days flew by as I was busy with research.

Was lovely to spend time with Harry and on Sunday night and Monday night, we watched X-men films, whilst drinking Horlicks. I have decided I rather like Wolverine!

On Tuesday evening, my friends who I worked with at Chester uni came round and we had a Chinese takeaway. Harry was very sociable and chatty and we all had a good evening. They helped me get Max's new wheelchair into the boot of my car, ready for bringing it to Newcastle.

Whilst I was away, Max went from strength to strength, gaining weight and feeling cheerful. It was lovely to see him again on Wednesday and although he was tired, he looked better than on Sunday. He did some maths with the hospital schoolteacher and tried hard with his physio, although his heart rate went up to 155 beats just with a bit of light on the spot marching, so he is very frail still.

His oxygen levels and adrenaline have been turned down a whisper, so that's good, but Paul and I both feel that it's unlikely that he will be let out of intensive care before a new heart comes. Reassuring in a way, as the nursing is one to one!

His oxygen tube was removed on Thursday morning as he was doing so well.

He had a busy day on Friday with an organised trip in his wheelchair down to the playroom and a trip to the shop to spend his pocket money. But this wore him out and by Friday evening, he had a bad headache and was exhausted. He fell asleep at 18:30 and woke again at 9:00 am on Saturday, other than a few medication wake-ups.

However, he had bad tummy ache, but this improved as the day went on. Had a lovely visit by brother, Dan, sister-in-law, Anne and niece, Rachel. We met at The Victory for lunch and then went to see Max (in shifts, due to the maximum numbers rule in PICU). Max loved seeing them and it did him a great deal of good psychologically. Later on, he started to get tummy ache again and then had a terrible vomit. Poor Max. He didn't even shed a tear. He just asked for a wet wipe and a back stroke! The docs were concerned as these are symptoms of heart failure, as the right side is still struggling. They adjusted some diuretic medication to help the flow of the HeartWare machine.

Again, I stayed with him whilst he slept and watched a DVD at his bedside.

By Sunday, he had bounced back and felt well enough to get dressed, so I washed his hair and body and he looked really spruced up. Back to Cheshire now. Love, Em X

"Hi, Emma – So good to hear that Max has had a better week. So many prayers and positive thoughts coming your way. You must be so proud of the way he is coping – what a little warrior. Let's hope that it won't be too long now before he wins his battle. Lots of love to you all, Gill and Lewis"

"Hi, Em, so glad to hear you have had some normality last week, albeit a small bit but worth it, I'm sure for you. If love and prayers were the answer to Max's health, he would be running out of the ward by now, fit for anything. We are all still behind Team Johnson, hoping it won't be too long before you have Max back home. As always, we send our love and you are all in our thoughts. Much love, Liz and Michael xxx."

"Thanks for the update, Emma, and so glad to hear Max had a better week. Have the (Irish) Catholics and (international) Buddhists praying for him – 106 of them yesterday! Thinking of ye all, Margaret xxx."

"Emma, I so look forward to your updates on a Sunday – what a great resource this is. I just want to say the afternoon spent last week with Max was such fun and he is my little hero – brave, independent, vulnerable and full of love. You can be so very, very proud of him! It was also incredibly encouraging to read of the progress that he is making – I can understand you were concerned about Friday, but so pleased that he bounced back by Sunday. He's heading in the right direction, Emma, so we'll keep praying and holding him in our hearts. Looking forward to catching up – much love to you all xxx, Norma."

"Keep going, Ems. One day at a time, each battle faced and overcome. Great to get the news. Much love to all. Nic xx."

DIARY OF A HEART MUM: Eighth Weekly Update – Sunday, 12 March 2017.

A great week! Max has been stable, perky and without any pain or discomfort. The most consistent week so far, in terms of a week without any emergencies or setbacks. Milrinone is still on 0.6, but the adrenaline came down from 0.04 to 0.02, then 0.01 and by Saturday, it was switched off! If on adrenaline, he has to stay in intensive care, so there is the possibility now that next week, Max might go back downstairs to the High Dependency Unit. I think Max's progress this week has surprised and thrilled the doctors and nurses. Quite unexpected! I'm sure everyone's thoughts and prayers have helped, along with Max's attitude and sense of humour!

I managed to go to work on Monday and Tuesday again. I am keeping happy with research. Harry was in Newcastle with Paul on Sun, Mon and Tues. Harry and Max were asking for each other. That, coupled with the bad day Max had a week last Saturday, meant that we let Harry miss two days of school. It was strange being in Rose Cottage all on my own, so I decided to watch a film: 'Arrival' – not the best choice of film in our circumstances. It wasn't the simple alien theme film that I thought it would be! It was very moving!

I arrived back in Newcastle on Tuesday night and I must have passed Paul and Harry coming back the other side of the motorway!

Three months since Max was admitted to hospital. Where has the time gone?

Max and I have had some great days together. We watched Trigger Happy TV, the Dom Joly comedy. Max was in stitches (mmm bad choice of phrase!) watching the giant telephone sketches. We took a trip in the wheelchair down to the playroom and he imagined his monitor machine was a large mobile phone and he pretended to answer the phone saying, "Hello... I'm in the playroom... Yeah... It's rubbish!" He had the nurses and play specialists laughing!

On Friday, Max had an appointment at the hospital hairdresser to have his hair cut. The nurse and I wheeled him along, complete with his battery pack and machinery for his HeartWare and his Milrinone IV. He attracts a lot of looks, as he has so much 'stuff' accompanying him, but he doesn't seem to notice or mind and likes saying hello to people.

Max's weight is now 22.8 kg, so fantastic weight gain! His appetite is really good too. His iron is very low, so he is taking extra iron, but that's straightforward.

He still needs that heart and I just hope it comes whilst he is so stable and strong, as this will help his recovery post-transplant. Max is sharing some worries and fears about the operation to come, so we are all working together to help alleviate these concerns.

Paul's Dad, Nigel, visited on Saturday. I showed him Scott House where we are staying and he was very impressed. Love, Emma XXXX.

"Glad to hear that things are on the up! Crossing everything I have for that heart to be available darling Em. Lots of love, Steve xxxxxx."

"So happy that you have positive news to relay. Such a relief after the alarming setbacks recently. Your life has been turned on its head, but you have created a new routine, which is now the norm for you. It's a great thing to be adaptable and able to adjust to new circumstances. Three months is a long time! My longest spell was

seven weeks and I was pretty institutionalised by then! Love and hugs to Max, and to you, Paul and Harry as well xxxx, Liz C"

"Great to hear he's had a much better week, sounds like he's back to his fun self – entertaining the nurses! Stay strong, Max, we are all thinking of you! Much love from all the girls at the Building Society xxx"

"Hi, Emma, it is absolutely wonderful to hear that Max has had a good week. As always, our thoughts are with you. Max is often mentioned by the Cubs as we sit together doing activities. Last Thursday, we all made boxes from card which we will decorate next Thursday and then we will fill them with chocolates for Mother's Day. All of the leader team have asked that I send their love and best wishes to Max and yourselves. Let's hope that Max stays well. Love, Bernard and the Over St John's leader team."

DIARY OF A HEART MUM: Ninth Weekly Update – Sunday, 19 March 2017.

Max got the go-ahead to be discharged from PICU and he moved downstairs back to the High Dependency Ward on Monday. Great news. Paul and I don't have to wear those awful plastic aprons! Ha-ha! Max has settled well into the ward and continues to do really well. He has been stable now for two weeks. They are keeping him on 0.6 Milrinone for now.

On Sunday evening, Harry and I had dinner with Chris and Avril, from St Chad's church. Delicious Lasagne! On Tuesday, Helen, Max's Godmother, and our neighbour, Neil, came over to help with the ironing. We ended up drinking rather than ironing…ha-ha! (Helen on Schloer!) But Helen and Neil both took a bag of ironing. Such gestures are amazingly helpful, as I'm finding it very difficult keeping on top of house jobs. So kind of them!

Drove back to Newcastle on Wednesday, and Paul and I met fleetingly at Wetherby Services for a 'handover'. It was lovely to see Max and he is doing so well, but he gets upset when his dressings are changed and is very nervous about his scar. He can get frustrated with his situation, but is coping remarkably well. We have a wheelchair trip once a day and travel around the hospital.

Max has a new friend, called Harry, funnily enough. They have playdates and x-box challenges together in the playroom.

By Friday, Max was brave enough to let the nurses remove the plaster on his chest scar, so that it would heal better with fresh air – fresh 'hospital air' that is!

Now that Max is so stable, I have had time to think about what the future holds. On Friday, I downloaded a Children's Paediatric Heart Transplant booklet from Great Ormond Street, full of useful information, but very daunting and sobering in terms of post-transplant prognosis and complications. Made me realise that post-transplant will be a whole new and challenging chapter in this sorry saga! Felt quite upset and depressed. I wandered along to the David Lloyd club for some tea and watched everyone with envy as they went about their normal lives, playing tennis, laughing with their kids, planning holidays. I wonder whether our lives will ever be 'normal' again. I stayed with Max whilst he slept, as I do on Friday nights and watched the film 'Elizabeth' with a bag of Maltesers. Long film, and I made my way back to Scott House at 23:00, stopping off at the hospital chapel to say a prayer. Felt upset when I spotted the Children's Heart Ward Memorial book.

Harry has been having nightmares recently, so the school counsellor saw him and will arrange sessions, which I hope will help.

On Saturday, Jacqui and Alex from Winsford Tennis Club travelled to see Max. We had lunch in The Victory and then joined Max in the ward. We played word games and puzzles and it was a lovely afternoon.

Drove back today. Missed my turn off after Wetherby whilst daydreaming and ended up somewhere near Ripon! Got back just in time to join Harry and Paul for lunch at Neil's house.

The lovely Norma dropped in to the ward today to see Max as he was on his own. Norma brought a fart whistle which Max loves! Just up his street! As I finish typing this, I am feeling really drained/exhausted. There just aren't enough hours when I am at Rose Cottage to get all the family paperwork/business jobs done etc. Still… nice to be home to see Harry, but just not seeing enough of Paul. We really are a fragmented family! Hopefully, I will feel a bit better next week.

"Emma, you're so brave to write all this down, it's a privilege actually to be party to your thoughts at this incredibly difficult time. Focus on your amazing family and how far you've come, and try not to look at other 'normal' families – we're all in abnormal situations *at some point in our lives (maybe not as extreme as yours, granted) – they might have had their trauma and come through it – as will you. Hugs and love xxxx, Fiona."*

"Your new normality has come so suddenly and has changed your lives so much. Thank you for sharing your thoughts and feelings so candidly. Nic."

"Oh, Emma – what you're all going through is bound to feel unreal, frustrating, unfair and absolutely exhausting! The fact that you find the strength to even share these updates with us is a clear indication of your incredible determination to not be beaten! That, along with your pure goodness and positivity and love, will see you through this bumpy and sometimes unpredictable journey and get you to your ultimate destination of a happy, healthy and together family again. Just make sure you remember to take good care of you too, lovely – your wellbeing is paramount. Sending big love, hugs and prayers xxxx, Maria"

"Your lives WILL be 'normal' again, but for the time being, what you have is normality, and all the focus is on Max's health. You would be very unnatural not to be thoroughly fed up at times. It's a stressful situation, yet you have to cope with it without the person you need most. It's very, very hard. But the good thing is that Max is stable and ready for the heart when one is available. And that's what all this is about. Your family may be fragmented but it's very strong as well. Perhaps you could have some counselling as well? It may help to pour it all out. You could show them your very clear and honest weekly blogs. Keep your chin up and sing whenever you can! xx. Liz C."

When we spoke with Dr Reinhardt in January 2017, the reality of our situation was necessarily laid out in sharp relief – all of the potential complications, life limitations and drawbacks were presented as the new reality we were facing. Underpinning this, though, was a very simple bottom line: without a transplant – an urgent transplant – Max would die. Be clear, there was no ambiguity here. The outcome was certain.

It is very hard not to become a Google obsessive, as you search to try and understand what you have been told. This is a personal decision, but one must take this course with care. Google has many articles and research papers relating to transplantation: survival rates, male/female matches, impact of heart rate on long-term outcome and so the list goes on. To truly understand the content, however, is a different matter altogether. One might read an executive summary or two, but the findings and the commentary around them are written for people who understand the complex medical terminology within and I didn't. I saw plenty – and I mean plenty – of living, breathing and indeed breeding examples of people living relatively long and happy lives with donor hearts, so why could this not be Max? Okay, it may not be, but why not? The point is, you don't know how it will pan out. Do any of us?

Prior to the invention of mechanical support, in the form of Max's HeartWare LVAD, the reality of the situation is that he would, more than likely, have died at some point during February of 2017. He was at imminent risk of death before the LVAD being fitted. Since the Millennium – very recent history by any standard – the outcome for Max had flipped from inevitable death by natural selection to one of hope. Who knows what will happen in the future, with the British Heart Foundation's 'T cell' research, stem cell research, mechanical hearts and the ability to grow organs for transplantation? It may be many years away, but the idea of mechanical pumps being fitted into the hearts of small children, the idea of transplantation itself, was considered the stuff of science fiction and far-fetched fantasy within the timescale of living memory.

It is hard to rationalise all of the emotions one feels about transplantation and the daily uncertainty of waiting for it to happen – if it ever happens – and the impact it has on you both personally and as a family. It is tempting for people to say 'You've just got to get on with life'. Whilst this is right and a truism that is not lost on us, it is a somewhat simplistic thing to say. When facing the current, known and most likely outcomes, it is incredibly hard and upsetting as a parent of a child who has just turned ten to know that, with near (but not complete) certainty, you will be burying your child. I have heard life with a transplanted child described thus: you have a clear blue sky above, but there is a cloud there – hopefully, only a small one – but it is there and it will never go away. This is the price you pay for knowing some tough, daunting and distressing facts that most of us, thankfully, do not need to know nor deal with.

DIARY OF A HEART MUM: Tenth Weekly Update – Sunday 26 March 2017.

NONE.

DIARY OF A HEART MUM: Eleventh Weekly Update –
Sunday, 2 April 2017.

Well… Two weeks since the last update. We were all hit by norovirus, except Paul, thankfully. Max was given IV fluid, but recovered relatively quickly. His Milrinone had been reduced from 0.6 to 0.5, but as expected, that didn't work and is now back up to 0.6 and likely to stay that way.

The ward has been on lockdown and as such, the nurses helped Max to build a cosy den in the next bed space, complete with 'Mystery Shack', 'No Doctors Allowed' and 'Max is the boss' posters. Whilst we have enjoyed some DVDs cuddled up in the den, Max is starting to get a bit of cabin fever – desperate for fresh air and walks, but trapped inside. On his walks to the bathroom, he stops at the window and gazes at the 'hosts of golden daffodils' on the other side of the glass. He says nothing but just seems to reflect (pardon the pun!). The weather in Newcastle has been pleasant, which makes it harder stuck on ward. Roasting in ward, and I can understand why Max gets hacked off! He is still very stable physically, so that it good news.

He has had a slight problem with his Alan Rickman Line (our made-up cockney Rhyming slang for Hickman Line), in his neck which is refusing to give blood. So, Max is back to needles for blood-taking for the time being.

We had to cancel visitors due to the lockdown, but there are quite a few visitors over the Easter Holidays.

Max enjoyed pranking the staff on April fool's Day. Plastic insects, pretend poo, nail through finger etc. etc. The old tricks are the best. Max's high spirited and positive demeanour can be deceptive and lull you into a false sense of 'wellness'. A quick glance at daily medical notes is a sobering reminder of his situation; phrases like 'End Stage Heart Failure', 'Milrinone dependent' and 'Urgent transplant list – awaiting transplant' jump off the page and hit you in the soul, reminding you of the gravity and cruelty of it all.

One of the nurses sat down with me and explained all the medication, as I don't have a clue what most of it is and what it is for. He has a total of 13 medications, including Milrinone! One of his medicines is for pulmonary hypertension, but it is, in essence, Viagra! This would explain why he is getting some eeerrr discomfort in the nether regions!

Harry now has an appointment coming up to check his heart and the GP needs to refer Paul and I through to the Manchester Heart Centre Inherited Cardiac Conditions Clinic for screening. More for peace of mind, I hope!

Harry is coping OK, but I really worry about him and sometimes feel that there is an emotional distance growing between us. Hopefully, it won't last!

Finally, thank you so much if you have sent a letter, card or gift. Please forgive us and don't take offence if we can't thank you for each and every gift. Sometimes, the generosity is overwhelming and when trying to juggle Cheshire/Newcastle and work/hospital, then it can be really hard keeping on top of who has sent what, especially if things arrive at the hospital whilst I am in Cheshire!

I have even had to set up a mini-office in the corner of Max's bed space to keep on top of work remotely, so struggling to find time to organise thank you cards. That said, we are of course, so grateful for kind gestures.

"Hello, Emma, lovely to get your update, but sorry to hear about the horrid norovirus. I am amazed at how you are managing to balance everything. It was good to read about the fun Max had on 1st April – it must really help him. Let's hope that you can have some quality family time this Easter and that Max continues to be stable. At Easter time, we think of new life and wouldn't it be a miracle if a heart became available at this time. With love, Gill and Lewis."

"Hi, Em, thanks so much for this latest update and glad that this nasty norovirus has gone. Something you could all have well done without! Thanks too for finding the time to keep us all informed in the hectic and worrying world which is carrying you along at the moment. We do all think and talk about you very often. Just sending you all our love as always and keep strong. Big hugs to Harry and Max (and to you and Paul of course!), Janis, Mike, Jenna, Alan and Karis xxxx."

"My, how I missed you! But you're back to fill us in on all your news. Well done, Max, on your "den". Oh wowee. You took me back 60 odd years ago when I built a den out of apple cartons in my back yard in a terraced house in Chesterton! No one was allowed in though, apart from 'Lobilob'. Now, Lobilob always shared any treats coming my way, like chocolate buttons or liquorice allsorts! They never ever saw Lobilob; strange that. Anyway, thank you for *all the news and to hear that Harry and Paul are well too is just a bonus. Take care. Love to all, Malcolm and Sue xxx."*

One would be forgiven for thinking that hospitals would (or at the very least should) be bug-free environments. We all know that this is not the case. That said, our experience at the Freeman was that it wasn't for the lack of trying on the part of the hospital, to minimise the likelihood of an outbreak of some description. Unfortunately, it doesn't take much to light the touch paper of an epidemic, the consequences of which, by definition, reverberate across the ward and wider hospital community.

It was a real bugbear (pun definitely intended) when people visiting the ward didn't wash their hands. A huge logo on the floor, signs on the wall and a sink right in front of you as you crossed the threshold, were clearly not enough for some people. Selfishly, they brought the risk of infection directly onto the ward, which was treating very poorly children – some immuno-suppressed – incredulously, some of them related to the offending soap dodgers.

So it was that the ward suffered an outbreak of norovirus. Poor little Max was unable to avoid this nasty invader; neither did his Mum, brother and most of the ward. High Dependency was in lock down and Infection Control, in their sharp crimson uniforms, were all over the problem like a rash (unfortunate choice of words!). Max, who suffered with a delicate tummy anyway, had the terrible discomfort of this all-encompassing virus to deal with. As one of the sufferers, he was placed in quarantine. Yellow tape was stuck to the floor around his bed space – as though an invisible force field to keep the nasty bug contained! Visitors were restricted to waving to him through the window and I had to wear plastic aprons, which made me sweat even more than normal.

Unfortunately, this particular outbreak (I recall there were two during Max's stay) coincided with Mother's Day. Emma and Harry were both confined to bed with severe bouts of this pernicious virus, so I was left to hold the fort with Max. Using some of his pocket money, Max had bought a little figurine of a mother, holding some flowers, from the tiny gift store at the front of the hospital. With Helen, his teacher, he had made a card to the 'Best mum in the World'. Unfortunately, these had to be delivered by me, but I recorded a video of Max wishing his Mum a happy Mother's Day and she reciprocated with a video of thanks.

It may not seem like much, but missing Mother's Day for Emma was a real blow. For her, it epitomised the sadness and sheer bad luck of our predicament – that she could not be with her precious younger son on a day intended to celebrate the bond between mothers and their offspring. It was made doubly hard because – although we didn't like to dwell on the fact – it could be the last Mother's Day she got to spend with Max. Although such thoughts were often repressed, the inescapable gravity of Max's illness meant that it was hard wired in our brains.

Incredibly, given his delicacy, Max bounced back quicker from this gastric gate crasher than either his Mum or Harry. After twenty-four hours, Max had started to feel more of sorts. Emma and Harry were still delicate when they returned to Cheshire, three days later. On this occasion, I was the last man standing; this bullet I managed to dodge.

DIARY OF A HEART MUM: Twelfth Weekly Update – Sunday, 9 April 2017.

Max has been really stable this week…but he does tire out by evening.

I was in Cheshire for most of the week. On Monday, my line manager told me that I had passed my probationary period! Don't quite know how I managed that under the circumstances, but this has given us some peace of mind. I celebrated with an Indian takeaway and a large glass of white wine, but felt strange on my own!

Paul and Harry have been in Newcastle whilst I worked. Max has had a really good week, although he still worries about the prospect of a feeding tube.

Harry seems more relaxed and he managed a fantastic school report despite all the upheaval.

The ladies in The Nationwide all clubbed together to put together a box of goodies for our family. Very kind and heart-warming! On Friday evening, I met with some friends in The Old Star Pub.

Drove back to Newcastle yesterday and met with Roger and Lucy and their three boys, James, Edward and William. We were able to take Max across the road in his wheelchair to Freeman Park and he walked round the pond and fed the ducks. He loved being properly outdoors, away from the hospital grounds for the first time in exactly four months. It was amazing to see. He was pretty exhausted by the evening, but worth it for the adventure. Jo, the play specialist, who is 'HeartWare' trained, joined us.

Max being so stable does make this easier for us, but the prospect of the big operation is never far from our minds. Alex from St Oswald's also visited us, which was a welcome change.

We went for another walk to the park this morning and the weather was glorious. There was a fun-run going on for charity. Said goodbye to Paul and Harry as they went back to Cheshire, making a stop at Mum and Dad's for dinner, and Harry is staying with them for a couple of days for a change of scenery.

A relative, Suzanne, sent a lovely wooden plaque, which has the following words on 'You don't know how strong you are until you have no choice but to be strong'. Very true words! Love, Em X

"Hi, Emma, it was so lovely to see you and Max on Tuesday. You are both extremely brave and an inspiration to us all. Max was an absolute joy and still had that cheeky grin that I remembered. It looked like you are both in very good hands, as all the doctors, consultants and nurses seemed very nice. I hope Max has another stable week. Alex."

"Hi Em, so glad that Max has had a more stable week, but realise that the same big worry is always with you. Well done on passing your probation period at work! I really don't know how you have kept going but the words on your plaque are very true! Hope you enjoy The King and I on Saturday! First night went well so fingers crossed for rest of week! Managed to get up off our knees from kneeling so all was well lol! Really looking forward to seeing you again when we can. In the meantime, much love as always to you all from us all xxxx, Janis."

"Good to hear you all enjoying the outdoors and sun, despite the horrendous situation. All our love, the Abbotts."

"What a brilliant week you've all had. Max must have been thrilled to get outside for a while, and well done, Harry, on your great report! Suzanne's words are very true, and you are all living proof of it! Take care, love from Jane and Bob x."

Being dependent on Milrinone, and after May 2017, Dobutamine as well, placed significant restrictions on Max's movements. Whilst the fitting of the LVAD afforded significantly greater freedom than the larger, more cumbersome Berlin Heart arrangement, Max's cocktail of drugs meant that we had to be accompanied by a nurse on any trips off the ward. As the doctors and nurses worked their miracles and stabilised Max's condition post his blip in the early spring, being able to leave the ward became extremely important to Max, as it represented a small but significant taste of independence.

That said, it required some logistical preparation. Firstly, his wheelchair – festooned with lights which spelled out his name, and flaming hubcaps no less – had to be fitted with two medication pumps; with careful twisting, these could be fixed to the handles of the chair, without hitting Max's head. Over the handlebars, we hung the HeartWare controller and batteries, as well as a spare controller and spare battery. Finally, we had to ensure that Max was clad in appropriate clothing – the North East can have some gorgeous weather, but then again…

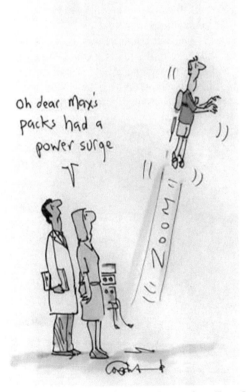

Cartoon sketched for Max by Private Eye Cartoonist – Tony Husband

So, we had Max and all of his paraphernalia, a parent to provide locomotion and a nurse just in case. Walks had to be worked around nurses' break time, which was no mean feat if the ward was busy. Occasionally, other children would join us, but mainly the walks were just for Max. First decision was which direction – along the Magnolia Mile to WH Smiths and the inevitable look at sweets, ear buds, headphones and negotiations about unpaid pocket money! – or out of the Cardiothoracic entrance and into the park area at the front of the hospital. To add a degree of spice, I would sometimes push Max around the corners 'taking' the bend on two wheels. Of course, to overturn would be disastrous and no doubt lead to much paperwork being completed by the accompanying nurse, but I was always careful to keep full control of the chair, even if I gave the opposite impression to Max.

Spotting certain 'landmarks' would be a key activity – and by 'landmarks', I mean things that had caught Max's attention on previous walks. A particular favourite was the abandoned bird's nest in a bush, situated close to the lower ground entrance in the older, tower block building. The incinerator, just along from 'Bird's Nest Row' was also of great interest, in particular, Max's fascination with how the chimney was constructed. Simple things.

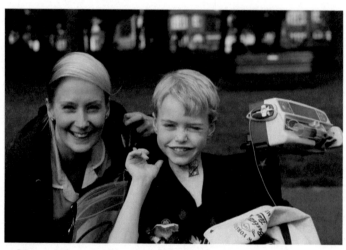

Max and Nurse Sophie, on a walk to the Freeman Park, opposite the hospital
Photo Credit: Marcus Taylor

These walks were made particularly special by two of the nurses with whom Max had developed a really lovely bond. Sophie – who was the nurse who drove to McDonald's after her shift to buy fries for Max – took the excitement to another level…quite literally. Now, for me, being built more for comfort than speed, the walks (scintillating cornering aside) were usually just that; taken at a walking pace. Sophie, however, as an experienced runner, upped the ante somewhat. Max would often, when traffic volumes on The Mile permitted, be seen heading off into the distance at a rate of knots, squealing with delight. By the time I had come level with the sharp left turn into the Institute of Transplantation, Max and Sophie were nowhere to be seen. Continuing at my normal and yes, somewhat sedate walking pace, I would be reunited with Max just outside the ward, being pushed by an ever so slightly flushed Sophie. Max would excitedly recount his journey, the details not dissimilar to the Monaco Grand Prix; tight turns and fast straights in a confined space! These little bursts of excitement really appealed to the side of Max's character that got him through this ordeal; the sense of fun and love of life, which refused to be extinguished.

Faye, who also occasionally took Max on his faster, shall we say expedited walks, also went the extra mile to keep Max's spirits up. Sydney was Faye's dog, and one afternoon, Faye took Max over to Freeman Park to meet Sydney, to have a walk and check out the duck pond. Faye had asked her boyfriend to bring Sydney to the park on his day off work, which he had duly done. Max was thrilled – he simply loves animals – especially dogs. Sydney was certainly not vicious (get it?), but she was a tad bonkers! A muzzle was in place, I think to protect her from herself! A proper livewire German Shepherd, Max adored spending time with her and it was such a thoughtful thing that Faye and her boyfriend did for the little man.

Walks also allowed Max the opportunity to develop his burgeoning skills as an amateur photographer. Max's Uncle Marcus – himself a keen photographer – had gifted Max his old SLR camera; a 'proper' camera with a big, professional looking lens. Max would take this camera on walks and would stop by an interesting bush or shrub, to take some close-up shots of leaves, flowers, water droplets and any attendant bug life inhabiting these spaces. Some of the resulting images were superb and beautifully detailed; Uncle Marcus had given Max some useful hints and tips and Max was proving to be a talented student. One of his photographs is included in this book. So long as we kept suitable control of his IV lines and HeartWare drive wire, taking these images again gave Max a very small but spiritually and psychologically important sense of freedom; he was, for a few minutes, truly escaping his plight and focusing on taking the perfect picture.

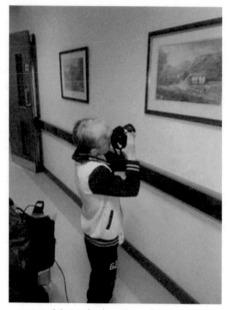

Max enjoying photography
Photo Credit: Emma Johnson

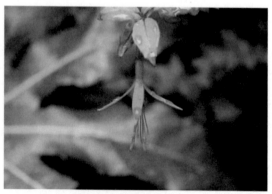

One of Max's photographs taken during a wheelchair walk
Photo Credit: Max Johnson

What we did notice on these walks were the looks from passers-by. Whilst to a degree, you become impervious to such occurrences, they did act as a stark reminder of Max's situation and how he must have appeared. At just over twenty kilograms, with pale skin and fair hair, Max looked what he was; frail. Add to this the fact that he was almost always in his wheelchair, accompanied by the IV pumps, controllers and batteries concomitant with his condition, then you can understand why people's attention was drawn to this little boy. One would think that this would be upsetting, but actually it wasn't. In just about every instance, the look was rooted in compassion and it didn't linger as though they were watching a freak show – it lingered just long enough to acknowledge the inherent sadness of the vista they were seeing, before a warm smile was directed either at Max or me and we moved on.

When you live in a hospital, dealing with such potentially grave conditions, you become accustomed to seeing people who are clearly in a battle for their lives, each one with their own stories of heartbreak. One prayed that there was also hope for each of them, but the reality is, this was not a universal state. Seeing people in this condition is terribly sad. Resting at the coffee tables in the café by the entrance to the hospital, underweight, drawn and frail looking, people would sit with their loved ones, IV machines next to them, and you would realise that personal suffering and tragedy is never far away. It comes to us all eventually. When that suffering strikes a child or young person, there is an extra sting in the tail to the cruelty of the situation and the shock and sadness one feels at seeing such a heartrending scene. To all of this, Max was largely oblivious – he was too busy soaking up his little taste of independence – that ability to say 'go left' and revel in the fact that we would do just that.

DIARY OF A HEART MUM: Thirteenth Weekly Update – Sunday, 16 April 2017.

We had a busy week this week, disinfecting and washing all Max's belongings in the post-lockdown deep-clean. Max was moved to a different bay temporarily, whilst a Hydrogen Peroxide Vapouriser machine was put in HDU for seven hours to kill off any remaining bugs.

We had a busy week with visitors. Mr Goodwin from Max's school came to visit Max on Tuesday, which cheered Max up no end. We went to the park for a wheelchair walk and fed the ducks. Went for lunch at The Victory!

On Wednesday, Charlotte, Harry's Godmother came to visit with her lovely son, Sammy. We spent some time in the playroom. On Thursday, Max's friend from St Oswald's, Jack, came to visit with his Mum and sister. By then, we were back in a new bed space in HDU, so could relax a little instead of living out of disinfected plastic bags! There are six bed spaces in HDU and Max has occupied all the spaces except one!

By Friday, Max and I felt quite exhausted. Sometimes it is hard putting on a brave face for visitors and afterwards, you can feel mentally very drained. Max had a funny turn in the bathroom when his face went beetroot red and he 'felt funny' with strong heart palpitations. His blood pressure went sky high and he couldn't breathe properly. It soon passed and he was OK. Max's LVAD had just been recalibrated, so the doctors think it was his body adjusting to the recalibration.

On Friday afternoon, Max felt recovered enough to prepare a magic show for the doctors and nurses (Thank you, Nationwide ladies, for the magic set). Max called himself 'Maxnificent, the Magician'.

Paul arrived in time for us to have tea together on Friday, and Max was thrilled to have both of us at the same time. Norma popped in briefly on Saturday morning, and Max recounted a very strange dream to us all. More like a nightmare!

I drove back to Cheshire on Saturday. Harry had a lovely time staying at his friend, Will's house. I picked him up and we headed home. I went to see The King and I at The Grange Theatre. It was a lovely show and great escapism. It was so nice to see friends from my musical theatre hobby.

On Easter Sunday, I was able to go to church with Harry for the first time since Max fell ill. It felt overwhelming and comforting all rolled into one. Our church friends are very lovely and caring! There was a little boy there who reminded me of Max! Back to work on Tuesday! Love, Em X.

"Lovely to see you on Saturday – your old smiley self. Great that you could see The King and I as well. It turned out to be a fantastic show. Let's hope you'll be back with us in a show in the not-too-distant future. Hope to see you for a longer chat soon. In the meantime, love and hugs for you both, and let's hope the spring will bring a 'new birth' for your brave little Max xx, Liz C."

"Hi, Emma, sounds like you've had an exhausting week! You need a lie down with a G&T! Thank you again for my visit on

Tuesday; it was fantastic to see how well Max was doing and what an amazing job you are doing keeping everything going! Visitors are nice – but it's also nice when they've gone and you can have a rest! Alex."

"Hi, Em, so glad to hear you've been 'released' from the lockdown. It's good to hear the news that Max is keeping his spirits up with doing the magic shows.

It was lovely to see you after The King and I production – so sorry it was so brief.

Big hugs for all of you. Stay strong. Penny, Nick, Zoe and Emily xxxxx."

"So lovely to see you, darling Em. You have a new fan in our Eve – she was absolutely besotted with you! Take care and hopefully, we will see you soon. Love to you all xxxxx, Steve."

We knew that Max's appetite was poor, so for Easter, instead of the usual chocolate egg, which we knew would gather dust or end up in the wrong mouth (mine!), we bought Max a 'Willow Tree' figurine, called 'Heart of Gold'. The 'Heart of Gold' sculpture was inspired by a young cancer patient, Scott Kristopher Innes, at Children's Mercy Hospital. Susan Lordi, the designer, wrote: "Scott's boundless and positive energy reflected on those around him, and as a result, good things continue to radiate from his spirit. His courageous spirit and kind smile showed me how one little heart of gold can continue to bring so much love, joy and comfort to others. It is my hope that this figure expresses the pure and honest affection between a child and those who love and care for him." Max was so thrilled with this gift that Emma felt compelled to write a thank you note to the Willow Tree company. Her missive read:

"My nine-year-old son, Max, is waiting for a heart transplant due to heart failure. He has been in hospital for over four months. He had open-heart surgery in February to fit a mechanical pump in his heart as a bridge to transplant to keep the blood pumping round his body. The pump contains gold. I chose the figurine as an Easter gift for three reasons: 1) it looks just like him 2) it reflects Max's heart of gold as he is always brave, kind and polite 3) he has real gold in his heart inside the mechanical pump. He loves it and will keep it forever as a reminder of how well he did overcoming this difficult chapter in his life. Beats an Easter egg! Thank you for designing such a beautiful piece. Love, Emma."

Emma didn't necessarily expect a reply and so when the following response arrived, she was moved to tears:

"Dear Emma, oh, what an inspiring story! Your Max declares perfectly what Susan intended for this special sculpture. You see, she designed it for a young friend who was battling cancer. Max, in his own wonderful way, carries on that battle for enduring love that lasts more than a lifetime. Max is our hero as well as yours, for he inspires us to always give our best to the things we undertake, no matter how challenging. Emma, Max now has his own heart of gold beating within him, but soon, he will have a heart more beautiful than gold. He will have the gift of life from another person; he will have the depth of love that few people ever have the opportunity to experience; most of all, he will have your love for his very long lifetime to come. His future, and yours, are bright with promise! We know that every day will be a joy, and that Max will accomplish great things. Whenever you and Max glance at your 'Heart of Gold' sculpture, please know that you have friends here who are delighted with your story and who pray for you all the time. With our appreciation, The Willow Tree Team."

A few weeks later, and another note arrived, this time from Susan Lordi, who had designed the 'Heart of Gold' piece:

"Dear Emma, I am catching up with emails…your note and photo of your handsome son, Max, caught my eye – and my heart. Thank you so much for sharing Max's brave story. His smile! I loved the photo. This is the best feedback an artist could have – and no one else can communicate the essence of life better than someone like Max. He is the wise one. And we get to learn from his resilience, bravery and determination to live life to the fullest. Thank you, Emma – and love to Max from all of us on the Willow Tree team. Susan Lordi."

Beautiful, inspiring words like this truly leave a lasting impression. Max received a lot of correspondence from well-wishers. We always read the letters and cards to him, as it encouraged him in his battle and helped him to understand just how 'well' he was doing for such a small boy. He was already making his mark on the world and he needed to know that. Of course, that 'Golden Heart' figurine would take on even more symbolism in the months to follow.

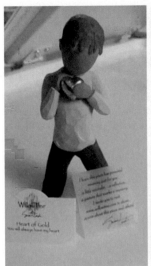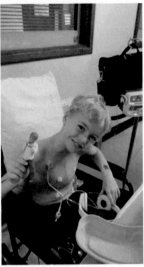

Willow Tree's 'Heart of Gold' Figurine
Photo Credits: Emma Johnson

Towards the end of April, Emma and I had managed to get a couple of nights away to celebrate our wedding anniversary.

To be clear about our ambition, it would have been quicker to walk back to the hospital than to drive, should we have been needed. Never mind, that isn't the point. What mattered was that we were going to have some time together, as a couple. We broke the news to Max that we were having two nights away, but stressed that we would pop to see him the following afternoon. By Sunday, we'd be back for good. Max's Auntie Anne, Uncle Dan and Cousin Rachel would be travelling from Leeds to spend all of Saturday with him, which was very kind of them. Nevertheless, Max was distraught at the prospect of his parents being in absentia. This would be the first time that we had been away (as stated, about 10 minutes' walk!) from him, and his reaction spoke volumes about how he had come to rely on us being there for him. It was like the separation anxiety one sees in a toddler, but on this occasion in a nine-year-old boy.

Emma was resolute that we should have some time together – she had a much better and more balanced approach to self-preservation than I. On the other hand, I was struggling to make the break and leave the ward, and I suspect that Max knew this and was working on the weakest link; me! He was in tears and complaining of feeling unwell. I was, not for the first time, like a defective motor, stuck between stators and thus unable to move. One of the doctors, Amelia, took us to one side. She could see that I was vacillating and that this, in turn, was causing Emma some distress. Amelia immediately reassured us; there was no clinical reason why we should not go. Yes, Max's position was of course precarious, but he was stable and we should not be cancelling our nights away based on any clinical concerns about Max. We must go. Amelia went and spoke with Max and reassured him, settling him beautifully, to a point where we were able to withdraw. As we left, she was sitting with Max, chatting away with him and he had really calmed. In the restaurant later that evening, my phone rang – it was one of the nurses – she was ringing to let us know that Max was fine and that we must enjoy our time away. How typically thoughtful.

This, however, was not the only act of kindness to come our way during our mini break. We had popped to the restaurant across the road from the hotel – the Pizza Express in Jesmond. We got chatting with the waiter; a student physiotherapist who was hoping to work on a placement at the Freeman. Our conversation inevitably turned to our circumstances, and the waiter listened intently as we explained our predicament. A short while later, he returned with our drinks and took our order. At this point, he announced that the meal and our drinks were on the house – the manager had been told of our story and they would be delighted to bestow this kindness on us. We couldn't believe it and both welled up at this simple, generous act. Living in two locations for such a long period is a significant hit to the finances, and our two nights away was a real luxury; this gesture really made the weekend and is yet another example of one of those acts of kindness and love that meant so much.

DIARY OF A HEART MUM: Fourteenth Weekly Update – Sunday, 23 April 2017.

This week, Max has been 'clinically stable' and in good spirits. One is constantly reminded of how vigilant the medical team is here. Earlier in the week, Max had a couple of disturbed nights with some heavy sweating. Those who know the Johnson family (and indeed the Lewis family – Paul's Mum) will know that there exists a propensity for sweating. However, it is also a sign of heart failure. As a result, not only did Max have the usual ward round visit by the doctors, he was also visited by the intensive care unit team…just a quick check on their part, but clear evidence they do not want to take any chances. Brilliant.

We visited – several times – the park opposite the hospital. This included a walk down to the waterfall…by far and away the greatest distance we've wandered from the hospital. Max loved it and played Poo Sticks on the bridge with his nurse.

We try to get out of the ward at least twice a day, which does take a little organising, due to a suitably trained nurse being required to come with us. However, Max loves this freedom and takes real joy in just being outside…and honking his wheelchair hooter! He also now propels himself along using his feet a la Fred Flintstone, and from a distance, he looks like a little raptor scurrying along the corridor!

Paul and I had Friday and Saturday away in a hotel in Jesmond, a belated celebration of our 15th anniversary. This was thanks to the Abbotts who looked after Harry and Dan, Anne and Rachel for looking after Max all day on Saturday. Max was distraught on Friday and had a terrible vomit just before we left. He didn't want us to go and we nearly didn't, but the doctors and nurses persuaded us that a break together would be a good idea and there was no medical reason why we shouldn't go. We reluctantly said goodbye and the nurse rang us to reassure us that Max was fine and had calmed down. So, we enjoyed a meal at Pizza Express. We had got chatting to the waiter, who is training to be a physiotherapist and he announced that the meal was 'on the house', a gift from Pizza Express, due to our circumstances with Max. We couldn't believe it and we both welled up with emotion. We wrote a thank you card and popped it in on Saturday. We went to Tynemouth on Saturday and got some sea air and the obligatory fish and chips!

My Mum has also been poorly lately. She was very ill this weekend with sickness and diarrhoea. She has been struggling lately and has been diagnosed with having calcified heart valves. More worries!

Today (Sunday), Max popped up to intensive care to meet a 14-year-old boy from Leeds, Connor. He had been admitted a couple of days earlier with exactly the same heart condition as Max. Surgeons are planning to fit a heart pump like the one Max has as a bridge to transplantation, and they felt it would be great for the young man to meet Max. Well, Max was lovely and was a real credit…we were very proud of him. Although we are in the midst of our own challenge, we both felt so strongly for the youngsters' parents…they were clearly still in shock. However, the boy's father stated that he felt very reassured after his chat with Paul. Whilst we pray daily for Max, we will do the same for them also.

During this meeting, the head surgeon came into the room. You could tell he was pleased to see Max, who was explaining how much more energy he had and that he was 'good to go'. With this, the 'Boss Man' turned to Max and gestured towards him, with a glint in his eye, telling him, "We haven't finished with you yet!" So sweet!

So, a week which demands positive assessment – Max's own heart is not going to get better – but the team here has worked wonders to get him to a position of relative stability. Whilst we will never take this for granted, nor expect it to last indefinitely, it certainly helps us to remain positive and hopeful that he will receive his 'little gift' and a chance at a normal life. Love to you all…

"Glad Max is enjoying the hooter on his wheelchair, told Gary and think he is very jealous and would like one too. You are always in our thoughts and prayers you are all so brave. Love you lots and an extra big smile from Gary x, Liz."

"Good to see so much positivity in your update, Emma, and how wonderful that Max can be a supporting influence on another young lad. Thinking about you and your family lots. Love, Jac and Jeff xxxx."

"Thanks for the update, Emma. So pleased Max is relatively stable, also that you and Paul managed a couple of days away. So sorry to hear about your Mum, I hope she's able to have her op soon and makes a full recovery. My thoughts and prayers are with you and your lovely family. Stay positive, lovely lady. Love, Paula xx."

"Hi, Emma, all this has been uplifting! It is wonderful that Max is unsurprisingly supporting others. Fantastic that you and Paul had time together too. Time is precious as you both know all too well. It's lovely that you can go out with Max too and do almost normal things. All looks well. Love to you all and to Harry too…congratulate him on excellent school results! Malcolm and Sue xxx."

Chapter 7

Throughout Max's time in hospital, we were asked to make numerous life changing, and as was our hope, lifesaving decisions, but there was a real risk that we would overlook Max's take on what was happening. It would be wrong to think that, just because we were wrapped up in carrying the responsibility of making these decisions, the whole process was not affecting Max profoundly and fundamentally. On one of the occasions that Max's spirits hit a very low ebb, we knew that something needed to be done.

Working with the psychologists, Kathryn and Sue and the play specialists Jo and Karen, we introduced Max to the 'Worry Monster'. This was a small green and purple stuffed monster with a large zipped mouth…remember Zippy? During the day, Max was encouraged to write his concerns down on a piece of paper, and then to place the paper into the Worry Monster's mouth. Burning the midnight oil, the Worry Monster would address Max's concerns with a hand written response to reassure him. It was remarkable how closely the Worry Monster's hand (claw) writing resembled my own and Emma's, but that was not the point – it allowed us to get an understanding of just what was on Max's mind that, perhaps, he didn't want to talk about directly.

Issues the Worry Monster addressed were at times hard to read – it gave a very real insight into how Max was truly feeling and just how well he had now gripped the reality of his situation. One of the first questions was 'Am I going to die?' Whilst the Worry Monster reassured Max that he was going to make it through this ordeal, the reality is we didn't have the answer to that question in a straightforward way – there was every possibility that he would die, but then if he received his little gift, the prognosis would be much better. Ultimately, the aim of the Worry Monster was to give us an insight into Max's deeper thoughts, so that we could do everything possible to lift his spirits during a particularly difficult time.

Occasionally, the questions would make us smile, even if we wouldn't wish to show approval to Max. Max was required to drink very high calorie apple flavoured drinks, which I can imagine felt like trying to squeeze a quart into a pint pot for his fragile tummy. Max simply asked the Worry Monster; 'Will I have to drink these ****ing drinks for the rest of my life?' Well, hopefully not, and the Worry Monster did ask Max not to swear, but his question had that feisty edge that told us there was fight in him yet. Some of the questions were truly considered, such as asking about medication post-transplant, and whether they would be liquid or tablets. All in all, the Worry Monster proved to be a very useful tool for us at a time when Max was feeling low and clearly had an awful lot on his mind that would otherwise have eluded us.

DIARY OF A HEART MUM: Fifteenth Weekly Update – Sunday, 30 April 2017.

This week, worked Monday and Tuesday. Completed interesting research, but been feeling very tired. I have to throw myself into the research to stop thinking about Max, but when I go for a break/lunch, it hits you like a monsoon!

Max has been clinically stable, but when we go for walks, we have to be very careful, as he does get out of breath. Max is sensible though and understands his own limits. Psychologically, this has been a tough week for all of us. The flip side of the position he is in is that Max is thinking about what he has to face ahead of him and the length of time (nearly five months) he has been in hospital is weighing heavily on his mind. We feel as though we are in the eye of the storm because we have had time to think about the enormous challenges that lie ahead, both in terms of waiting for the transplant, the transplant itself when it comes and the post-transplant recovery and adjustment period. The waiting is really tough, as we are in limboland/groundhog day, but with the Sword of Damocles hanging over us.

We have been struggling to encourage Max to drink his time-allocated swigs of special calorie rich apple juice and to get him to eat enough to gain weight. The frustration of this really got to me this week and I admit to bursting into tears in a meeting with the gastro/dietician team. The feeding tube still dangles in the background, waiting to pounce! Had a good chat with the psychologist about this and she feels that the frustration and near-obsession/fixation with Max drinking enough apple juice is symptomatic of the general frustration with this whole situation and a recent pessimistic and negative feeling that our lives will never get back on track!

I really enjoy reading about everyone's activities on Facebook, but there is a tinge of envy, as I just want our family to get back to a 'normal' life, whatever 'normal' is! Harry was distraught on Wednesday morning before going to school, as he was missing Max so much and couldn't understand why this has happened to us. I rang the school and the counsellor had a nice chat with Harry and he seems back on track.

Max has a worry monster cuddly toy. The play specialists encourage him to write any worries on a piece of paper and put it in the worry monster's zip up mouth. The monster digests the worries and in the morning there is a written reply (by us!). After not using it for a while, Max has used it a lot this week and his worries range from "I don't want to die" and "Will I ever go home?" to "Will my medicines after I have a new heart be horrible?" and, "When can I stop drinking this F*****g apple juice?" I think we can forgive him an occasional unspoken swear word.

Max and I were visited by Milly, my friend, Liz's daughter, who is a student living in Jesmond. She offered to pop in and visit Max and I. We had a lovely time and Max really liked her. Such a lovely young lady, with a great future ahead of her, I'm sure. That visit cheered us up. Met with Norma at The Victory on Friday evening and as usual, the time whizzed by, as we always have stimulating conversation. Norma popped in to see Max on Saturday, and brought a lovely healthy lunch for us, and watermelon ice bites for Max. Yummy! Max made some fudge with the play specialists and he really enjoyed cooking.

Harry and Paul arrived back on Saturday night, but Max had a big vomit, as he had eaten his tablets too quickly on the back of Domino's chicken wings. He is so brave when he is sick. His tummy is quite delicate due to his condition, but he bounced back very quickly and we went into the playroom and all watched Britain's Got Talent on the big screen. Max loved it, especially the magician!

Sunday was a good day and we took Max for a walk around the park pond and then popped into the David Lloyd Club for a cup of tea. Max was able to watch a game of tennis, but there were a lot of young children who were looking at Max curiously, due to his wheelchair, wires and machinery. All those healthy children and poor little Max. What a contrast! Max returned to have a syringe water-fight in the playroom garden with Faye, his nurse. He loved it, but got quite out of breath.

I am really hopeful that Max will get a new heart by the end of May, as this could mean going back to school in September. BUT, I mustn't raise my expectations, in case this doesn't happen and I will only feel dejected and disappointed. Of course, it's never far from our mind that Max will benefit from another family's tragedy!

"Hi, Emma. Thank you so much for the update. It's good that Max is continuing to be stable. The worry monster is a wonderful idea. It can be so difficult voicing your worries so to be able to write them and get assurance from the monster must really help. Who cares if the odd swear word creeps in. Five months is such a long time and let's hope and pray your wishes for the end of May are realised. It's good to hear that Harry is getting support. He must miss Max so much. With love, Gill and Lewis."

"Thanks for the update, Em. Feel free to pop in anytime on your Cheshire stints. Always good to see any of you, so please call in, even just on the off chance we are in. Always good to have a cuppa and a chat. Nic."

"Emma, you are an absolute gem writing this each week. I can't tell you how much it means to us to share a morsel of what is happening. Each week as the weekend approaches, we wait for the update to arrive! Thank you. You are all so incredibly brave and courageous, anxiously waiting for that step into the unknown. Max is an inspiration to us all and you must try to tell him, how he is affecting us all so positively. Our love to all of you. Xxx, Malcolm."

"You've just made me laugh and given me light relief from my maths planning with the 'When can I stop drinking this Fu…ing apple juice?' comment! Tell Max, I hope he has got his grammar the correct way in this sentence! Alex X."

Max had been fitted with a Hickman Line when he first had his LVAD operation. Essentially, a tube was inserted into his artery on the upper right side of his chest. This allowed Max to receive his intravenous drugs through this line rather than through a cannula on the back of his hand or in his arm. Unfortunately, after some time, the Hickman line stopped working and it was decided that another would be inserted, this time on the left side. Whilst this was a positive thing for Max, as it avoided the need for an unreliable and uncomfortable cannula, it still had to be undertaken with a general anaesthetic. I accompanied Max into theatre with one of the play specialists, Karen, and saw his eyes glaze over as the anaesthetic took him from the conscious world.

Luckily, the procedure went well, so we went upstairs to collect Max some two hours later, feeling relatively optimistic, if cautiously so. As I entered the recovery room, Max was crying and clearly in a lot of pain. The surgeon was doing her best to calm him, but he was having none of it. He looked at me, his big blue eyes full of tears and hurt and said, "Why didn't you tell me it would hurt this much?" His sense of betrayal was unmistakable and the crying consumed him once more. I was lost. I felt so guilty, helpless and useless that I could not do anything to help take this suffering away. His hair was matted to his head with sweat and he looked as white as a sheet. It was at this point that Karen – sensing my paralysis – stepped forward and started to soothe Max. She said exactly the right things, and although Max is headstrong and not often for turning, she managed to get him to calm down and relax. Back in the ward, I picked my little boy off the theatre trolley and with all the gentleness and love I could command, I put him carefully into his bed, where he lay motionless, eyes closed and lips pursed, trying to come to terms with and overcome his pain. To his credit – and not for the first or last time – he did. Thank goodness, once again, for the play specialist.

DIARY OF A HEART MUM: Sixteenth Weekly Update – Sunday, 7 May 2017.

On the morning of Bank Holiday Monday, Max had a bad swelling on his neck. It turned out that his Alan Rickman Line (Hickman Line) was blocked and the Milrinone heart drug was not getting to his heart... Max's right side of his heart is completely Milrinone dependent. Max explained that his neck had been hurting for three days, but he decided not to tell anyone! We explained to Max how important it is to let us know if he is feeling any discomfort or anything unusual. The blockage could explain why Max had the big vomit a week last Saturday and why Max's appetite has gone downhill (heart failure symptoms). The doctors stopped the Milrinone and the swelling gradually went down and they put a temporary cannula in Max's arm (he's so brave with needles) so that the Milrinone could be continued. He improved a bit, but had a funny turn on Tuesday morning when he felt unwell in the bathroom. We think it was because he had been standing for 20 minutes.

Harry has been so worried about his brother, but his school has been absolutely wonderful and so compassionate under the circumstances. We feel blessed that he goes to such a fantastic school.

This week, Max had his first shower since 1st February! This is because he has been provided with a special waterproof double layer bag for his machinery. He absolutely loved his shower and squealed in delight!

I went to work Tuesday and Wednesday and coped quite well. I am glad that people don't gush and let me get on with my job, but on the other hand, it would be nice if my neighbours at work would occasionally ask how Max is or how I am. I suffer in silence!

On Wednesday afternoon, Max had a general anaesthetic to have his old Hickman Line removed and a new one put in on the other side. He was gone over two hours and I had to wait it out at work, which was tough! He had a very sore, fragile and angry couple of days after the procedure, but at least the Milrinone is now getting safely to his heart again. We have been struggling to ensure that Max has enough fluid and food and it is stressful for everyone, especially Max, with all the pressure I feel we put on him. It distracts from having quality time together. It came to a head when at 4 o'clock on Friday morning, Max's HeartWare alarmed with a 'Low Flow' warning. This is due to not taking in enough fluid, so they gave him a fluid bag IV and the decision has been made that he will be fed through the Hickman Line from Monday and so he can eat as much or as little as he wants, without any nagging or fussing. However, drinking enough fluid will still be very important. This will take all the worry and pressure off, despite other risks.

On Saturday morning, Max had really bad tummy ache, which Calpol wouldn't shift, so they gave him morphine, which stopped his tummy ache, but made him a little 'spaced out' and 'hyper'. He insisted on wiping the doc's arm, ready for the doctor's cannula! He's trying to get his own back!

Mum, Dad and Marcus arrived for a visit on Saturday afternoon. We went to a lovely Italian restaurant 'Bistro Neri' in South Gosforth and then watched Britain's Got Talent in the playroom with Max.

Arrived back shattered on Sunday, for a quick handover with Paul but lots to do for work and other household paperwork. Until next week… Love, Em X.

"Another difficult week for all of you. You are all so brave the way you're dealing with everything life is throwing at you at the moment. Keep strong. Had a Pet Service at church on Sunday – it was amazing! As well as all the dogs that came along there was a rabbit, a hedgehog, a hamster…and a giraffe! (a massive stuffed toy, of course!). It was all great fun. Our love and prayers are with you all. Jane and Bob xx."

"What a very tough week you have all had. You truly are an inspiration to all. My kids are grown but a parent or family never stops feeling the anguish of their children. It is tough being a parent. You are all in my prayers as you face all that life throws at you. Send love to all please and if you don't feel brave, tell somebody and have a good cry. 'This too will pass'. Please tell Max he is a super star. Love and hugs, Auntie Wendy xxxx."

"You continue to amaze and inspire me, darling Em – how you function whilst dealing with all of this is beyond me. You are all so very brave. Steve."

DIARY OF A HEART MUM: Seventeenth Weekly Update – Sunday, 14 May 2017.

I am going to start this update about Harry. He and good friends/neighbours, Neil and Jennifer, will be doing a 5K run in July. Neil will also be doing an open water swim across Lake Derwent. These events are to raise money for The Sick Children's Trust which funds our hospital accommodation, Scott House, in Newcastle. It pays for other hospital accommodation facilities all over the UK too. An amazing charity which has helped our family enormously, by giving us a comfortable place to stay for over four months now. Harry and Neil have already hit 50% of the 2000 pounds target.

Alex Goodwin, Principal at Max's school (who visited Max in Newcastle) is also running 10k in a couple of runs to raise money for the same charity.

To Max: On late Monday, Max's liver was 4 cm enlarged and so his Milrinone has been put up to 0.7. The TPN food bag is going in through his new Hickman Line and so his blood is a little thicker than doctors would like and so he is having injections in his thigh daily to help to thin the blood. But Max is thriving psychologically and has been on excellent form this week. The nutrition through the Alan Rickman Line seems to be giving Max stacks of energy. P.S: New cockney rhyming slang: Milrinone = 'moan n groan' and TPN = 'Mother hen'!

On Thursday, Liz and Michael, our good friends from Yorkshire spent the day with Max. Liz, Michael and the nurses took Max for a picnic in the park and he had a lovely day. Thank you, Liz and Michael!

On Friday, Chris, our vicar from St Chad's Church in Winsford, travelled all the way from Cheshire to see us. We met at The Victory Pub for lunch and then spent the afternoon with Max. We played games and a good time was had by all. Chris showed Max some pictures and video of the recent Pet's Service at church. Speaking of pets, one of the nurses, Faye, brought her German shepherd puppy to the hospital on her day off to show Max. Max was delighted!

On Saturday, Max was the only patient in HDU, so we shut the blinds, put the disco lights on and had a disco, with Max as the DJ/mixer! Very warm in there though!

Max also has a new hobby, as Marcus gave Max an old camera that he doesn't use anymore. Max is taking photos everywhere he goes and just loves it! So nice to see him taking joy in the smallest leaf/insect/petal! I think we will organise a photo scrapbook for Max to look back on when he is through the other end of all this.

I drove back to Newcastle today (Sunday) and had a quick handover with Paul. Lovely to see Harry looking so bouncy and happy. The fundraising is helping him to cope, and I suppose we have all got used to our unusual and unexpected circumstance. Love, Em XXXX.

"Lovely to hear that Max has had a good week and found a new hobby. We shall certainly sponsor Harry and Neil – what a marvellous charity providing accommodation for families to enable them to be near their children in hospital. Don't know how you are managing, Emma. Keep hoping and praying to get that message to say Max has a new heart – let's hope it is very soon. Love, Gill and Lewis."

"Great to hear that Harry is more upbeat. I shall certainly donate to such a fabulous cause and the lads make their target. Good news too that Max has found something to do that he really likes. Photography seems to run in the family. Uncle Norman, (Way back!). Your Dad, my Dad, me, Sherri, Claire all love to take pictures, with some success and pleasure. I am in awe of all your *lovely family. God bless and keep you all in the palm of His hand. Lots of love and hugs. Wendy xxxx."*

"Hi, Em, thanks for your update! Lovely positive news, despite Max's physical problem this week. Well done to Harry – what a star he is! We have sponsored them. Also well done in advance to Neil and Alex! Great that Max is enjoying his new hobby – maybe this will be his career of choice? Much love to you all, as always xxx, Janis."

"Hi, lovely to hear about your news this week, and to hear that Max is getting a bit more energy. I loved his photos on Facebook, he is very talented! Also, a great thing he can do as he continues to wait in Newcastle. We have sponsored Harry for the race, just wish we had a few thousand spare as I would hand it over in a heartbeat to such a fabulous charity. I have seen Scott House and know just what a great place it is for you, and how it has made your lives so much easier in such difficult circumstances. Let me know if you fancy a chat this week. Take care, sending HUGE hugs and loves to you and your boys xxxx, Charlotte."

DIARY OF A HEART MUM: Eighteenth Weekly Update – Sunday, 21 May 2017.

I attended a peaceful church service on Sunday evening at St Chad's Church, which was lovely and very calming.

Managed work on Monday/Tuesday and threw myself into more market research.

Harry had his parents' evening on Thursday, and despite a little bit of inevitable absence due to our circumstances, he got good reports and the staff team were lovely.

Paul arrived home for a well-earned rest and Harry and I travelled to Newcastle together and arrived around midnight. We had a lovely day with Max on Friday. In the morning, Max was wheeled to Scott House to help to welcome some Royal Navy Sick Children's Trust fundraisers who had taken on an 'any which way' challenge to blag their way from Plymouth to Newcastle. They turned up in a police van with the sirens going. They had met some very kind folk along the way who had helped them on their long journey. They did it in one week. Max took some photos, but he said afterwards that he had felt a bit sad that he couldn't run around like the other children.

On Friday afternoon, there was a movie afternoon in the playroom. We all watched MOANA curled up on beanbags.

However, Max took a turn for the worse on Saturday and Sunday. His heart rate was going extremely high, he had backache, breathlessness, vomiting, diarrhoea and his face looked pallid with pale skin and lips. He had two very bad nights with little sleep. Very worrying and he can't eat anything. He was too breathless even to have a shower, so we had to leave him with matted hair. The doctors at first thought it might have been a kidney infection, but concluded on Sunday afternoon that these were further symptoms of heart failure, as the function in the right side of Max's heart had got worse.

A serious conversation was had with the doctors, who said that they would add a new IV heart drug called Dobutamine in addition to Milrinone and that they would up the Frusemide diuretic. By 16:00, when Harry and I set off to return to Winsford, Max seemed to have improved, but still, a real worry. The doctors mentioned that if he doesn't improve, then a Berlin heart machine might need to be considered! This would be very risky and we pray that this could be avoided.

So, a worrying weekend, and the next 48 hours will be very important to understand how Max is responding. Feeling deflated and exhausted. The prospect of getting up at 6:00 am for work is not one I relish tonight. Love, Emma X.

"Thanks for keeping us updated, Emma. It must be very hard for you to write these bulletins. Our thoughts are with you as always. Stay strong, you are so brave. All our love and best wishes to you all, Penny, Nick, Zoe and Emily xxx."

"I've not stopped thinking about Max today. Hopefully, he will continue to improve. Xx, Clare."

"Hi, Emma. Not a good week this one and so hard for you all. For so many of us far away, we do thank you for your weekly updates. We are all like a nightingale that is so small, you can hardly see it up there, high in the sky, yet it fills us with beautiful birdsong. You may not see us, Emma, but we are always there with you. Love to Harry, Paul, to you and wonderful Max xxx, Malcolm."

"Oh, Emma, how difficult and stressful for you. The worst possible thing – seeing your child in all this pain and trauma. Thinking about you all the time and wishing I could do something useful to help. Sending all our love xxx, Fiona."

"Emma, I so look forward to your updates, so thank you so much for making the effort to write these and send them out every Sunday. What a week this one has been for you all and I'm so very

upset to hear that Max has taken a turn for the worse. I didn't really know the implications of a Berlin heart machine but have done some reading on Gt Ormond Street Hospital website – I do get totally that we just want that new heart to arrive so that the focus is on recovery rather than stabilising and waiting – apart from the trauma of more interventions for you all. I'm holding you all in my prayers and meditations – much love to you, Paul and Harry, and I will be holding a very special place for Max and sending as much healing energy and love as I can muster. Emma, if there is anything at all that you or Paul need or I can do for you this week, then please do let me know as I shall be around! Much love and sleep tight – a good hot bath before you go to bed might help. xxx, Norma."

DIARY OF A HEART MUM: Nineteenth Weekly Update – Sunday, 28 May 2017.

The new heart IV Dobutamine, really seemed to do the trick and since Monday, Max has been stable again, if a little fragile. Conversations around possible Berlin heart machine have ceased, fortunately.

For the time being, he is not allowed to the park, but is allowed walks to the hospital garden and hospital grounds. The feeding through his Hickman Line doesn't seem to be helping Max gain weight, and in fact, he has lost weight, so there is a chance he will have to brave a feeding tube through the nose on Tuesday – under sedation this time! That's going to be tough! Max is on fine form, psychologically, this week, but we are worried that a feeding tube will set him back.

BBC 2 visited Max and Paul this week, as they are doing a documentary about heart transplants and they would like to follow Max over six months. This will include filming the transplant! Eek. Paul and I both think that this would be good to raise awareness about dilated cardiomyopathy and the symptoms, but also raise awareness about organ donation issues.

Max is back in his favourite spot on HDU, the corner of the ward where he landed when first admitted. By a window and more space.

Found it hard to drag myself to work last Monday and Tuesday after such a difficult weekend, but just about managed it. Was deeply saddened about the Manchester atrocity and it has preyed on my mind all week, as it has most people.

I travelled to Anglesey for a mini break alone. Stayed in a gorgeous B&B, the Castellar, in Camaes Bay. I tried to relax and I paddled in the sea and watched the sunset go down over the bay, with a cold glass of apple cider.

Drove back on Friday and in the evening, I went to watch Avenue Q at Northwich Memorial Court (Knutsford Musical Theatre Company). There was a page in the programme dedicated to Max and The Children's Heart Unit Fund, which provides ward equipment, play specialists and they also helped to raise money for Scott House. After the show, cast members collected donations in buckets from audience members. Very touching. This whole episode with Max's illness has made me realise and appreciate just how many friends I have made in musical theatre over the years, in Knutsford Musical Theatre Company, Mid-Cheshire Musical Theatre Company, Vale Royal Musical Theatre Company and Sale and Altrincham Musical Theatre Company.

I set off for Newcastle at 22:30 after the show finished and arrived at 2:00 in the morning. Very tired, but good journey. I knew it was the witching hour, as I found myself listening to The Shipping Forecast on Radio 4 (Cyclonic...Variable etc.)!

Had a great day with Max on Saturday and today. He was on really good form. We went for a nice walk around the hospital and Max took some lovely photographs. He might not be getting much of a school education, but he is learning in other ways, about photography, medicine, interacting with adults etc. The ward is full, so quite noisy, but we are used to that now. Have stopped anticipating a phone call about a new heart. Just taking it one day at a time. Love, Em X.

"Hi, Emma... I know that Paul and Harry are up at the moment so I hope that brings some light relief with the whole family being together. I am glad Max is stable once more and the talk of the Berlin machine has died down, and he is psychologically well. As always – love and best wishes to you all. Alex X."

"Hi, Em, thinking about Max today and hoping that he doesn't have to have a new feeding tube, and if he does, that it's not too stressful for him and you. So many ups and downs for you all. We're continually amazed by your strength, all of you. Thanks for all your news, and of course all our love. Janis, Mike, Jenna, Karis and Alan xxx."

"What a week again, Emma! It's a little like the magical mystery tour for us...so many twists and turns, and right in the *middle is magical Max. As always, we all send our love to you and hope that there will be good news around the corner. Love to Paul and Harry. Malcolm."*

"Dear Emma, glad to hear things looking slightly up for Max this week. Well done on actually doing any work. Mind yourself. Reading your posts has made me sign up to be an organ donor on my new (UK!) licence. I have my fingers crossed and other people praying that Max gets his heart soon. Hang on in there – you're all doing brilliantly. Much love, Margaret xx."

Prior to Max falling ill, I had not really appreciated or properly understood just what a pivotal role charities play at a local and national level in shaping and delivering care. I feel somewhat ashamed of myself now, for something which seems so obvious – more opprobrium coming my way. Charities really do work hand in glove with the medical professionals in the NHS. I now recognise just how much we rely upon this symbiotic approach to treatment, support and advancement.

Local to Newcastle, there is the Children's Heart Unit Fund, which does so much for the care of children with poorly hearts at the Freeman Hospital. Scott House, our accommodation, providing a home from home, is part of The Sick Children's Trust, which has similar wonderful locations at key hospitals across the country. Then you have the British Heart Foundation, without whom Max would not have had a transplant at all. They were instrumental in turning heart transplantation into an accepted treatment for those for whom the options had run out.

Looking to the future, the British Heart Foundation is funding research into improving the long-term outcome for transplanted patients. If you have a transplant at, say fifty, then you could reasonably expect, with good fortune, to make it to the biblical three score years and ten. If you have a transplant at nine, then this is not going to happen. That said, if the British Heart Foundation and their highly talented team of professors and researchers have their way, then such miracles may just start to become within touching distance.

It has been a privilege for our family to play a part in raising awareness of the work of the British Heart Foundation. Max was involved in the publicity surrounding the announcement of funding aimed at improving our understanding and treatment of cardiomyopathy – in its myriad forms. This disease was responsible for nearly taking our son from us, and brings such heartbreak to families as a silent, unseen killer, waiting in the wings for its ominous, devastating entrance. We will continue to support the British Heart Foundation in any way we can; we have so much to thank them for and they may yet be the key to improving the long-term outcome for Max. All power to their elbows.

So, whether it's providing practical support for patients, parents and practitioners on the ground, or pushing the boundaries of what is possible, charities are at the heart of supporting heart patients and their families.

DIARY OF A HEART MUM: Twentieth Weekly Update – Sunday, 4 June 2017.

So, quite a good, varied week. I booked the week off work, so was able to spend a full week in Newcastle.

Max is still very stable on the new heart drug and has made some new friends, one little girl who is waiting for a second heart transplant in 18 months! I really hope that when Max is lucky enough to be offered his 'gift of life', that his body will cope.

This week, the English Youth Ballet performed for the ward children in the playroom – Swan Lake. Very moving and quite ironic… 'The Dying Swan!' Max appeared on Look North TV, as he watched in awe, but there was an air of sadness as he looked on! What must he be thinking?

The production company for BBC 2 started talking to Max and filming him. However, he might not be featured if he doesn't get his heart by the end of July. On the other hand, it would make a strong point about waiting times for organ donation. So, we'll see. Other adults and children will be featured too. The directors are very sensitive and understanding about the situation our family has found ourselves in. They will just pop in occasionally for catch-ups and filming.

On Wednesday, Paul and Harry joined us and we have had some lovely rare family time together. Max has been loving Britain's Got Talent in the live semi-final/final week. On Friday, Harry celebrated his 12th birthday. The play specialist helped Max to make a 'Happy Birthday' banner. We had a pizza party with Max, and then in the evening, we took Harry out to Bistro Neri in South Gosforth for an Italian meal.

Yesterday, I took Harry to Blackpool for some quality time together. Today, we spent the day at The Tower, and went in the Tower Dungeon, up to the top of the Tower and watched the Tower Circus. The last time I was there was 33 years ago with my Granny

Muriel. She used to take me away occasionally to the Blackpool Butlins Metropole Hotel. We got through some 'Cinzanos and lemonade', I seem to remember! I was only just a teenager! Ha ha!

After the Tower, Harry and I took the tram back to Bispham and paddled/waded in the sea. Big waves and we got soaked. But what a good laugh we had together! The beach was deserted and the weather was perfect, and I even caught the sun. We walked barefoot back to the accommodation, getting some funny looks.

Roger, William, Edward and Gramps visited Max and Paul on Saturday in Newcastle. They had lunch in The Victory before seeing Max. Paul said they had a nice time.

So, a great week overall, but was very saddened to hear about yet another terror attack, this time in London. What is the world coming to!

"Hello, Emma. Thank you for the news that seems a little better this week. It's good that you have managed to get together as a family and enjoy being together. Sue, J and I go to Blackpool Tower on Sunday for a celebration of Phil Kelsall's years on the Wurlitzer. We love it in the ballroom…it is quite majestic. Glad that Harry and yourself had a special time together. Love to marvellous Max, Paul and Harry and to you. Xxx Malcolm."

"So good to read your update this week, it must have been great for you to have had time together as a family and particularly good for you to have had a special time with Harry in Blackpool. The Tower holds so many childhood memories – I never got to sample Cinzano. Good old Granny. As you say, the BBC programme will do so much good to highlight the need for donors, but let's hope and pray that Max will receive his before July. With love, Gill and Lewis."

"Hi, Em, so glad it's been a better and more positive week for you all! Belated happy birthday to Harry, and Blackpool sounded fab! Had a little giggle at the thought of you and Granny Muriel downing Cinzanos and lemonade! Hope you and Harry stuck to the lemonade! Take care, and lots of love as always xx, Janis."

"Glad to hear Max is more stable and great that you and Harry got to Blackpool, it's a great place. We love the Tower. See you soon once Rachel is back from Sheffield – where has her first year gone? Love, Dan and Anne xx."

Chapter 8

DIARY OF A HEART MUM: Twenty-First Weekly Update – Sunday, 11 June 2017.

Max has had another great week. I don't know what's in that Dobutamine, but it's got some kick! Max has been energetic, not tired, able to walk a lap of the hospital for the first time, and no breathlessness. Plus, he has been really witty and extra cheeky. If he could stay like this until a new heart comes, then the whole situation is much easier to cope with. He has been in hospital over six months now.

On a more sobering note, the medical team are definitely planning to put a feeding tube down Max's nose into his stomach on Thursday. This is going to be managed very carefully with the whole team (psychologist, doctors, consultants and gastric team) involved. It will happen under sedation, but the chances are that Max will kick off when he is told by the head honcho and then go into a depression like last time. However, the psychologist has assured me that it is a fear, rather than a fact! He might be OK! Unfortunately, feeding through the Mother Hen (TPN) line isn't working and Max is just not gaining weight. Although he is on great form, he does look visibly thinner, with his driveline cable protruding under his skin.

I worked on Tuesday and Wednesday and made my way to Newcastle on Thursday. The HDU ward is full to capacity, but the new quiet time from 14–16 is wonderful and allows downtime for everyone, without interruptions. The play specialists continue to do an incredible job and this week, they organised a quiz and also, Max had the wondrous experience of watching the caterpillar chrysalis turn into butterflies (Painted Ladies). The team also helped Max to decorate his wheelchair. He looks very cool on his wheelchair walks. They are obviously fond of Max and Max is fond of them.

Max's teacher, Helen, who teaches him one hour a day, sat down with me on Friday and showed me all his workbooks. I was so impressed with what he has managed to do in highly restrictive circumstances and the teacher has formed a wonderful bond with Max. We are so grateful to Mrs Bentley for collaborating with the teacher, so that Max is following the school curriculum, as far as is possible and as far as he is able. Very reassuring, but with no pressure on Max!

On Saturday, I had more HeartWare training and I was taught what to do if the full alarm goes off and how to change the controller if the controller fails and the mechanical pump in Max's heart stops working. The sister taught me on a pretend machine and I couldn't believe how loud the alarm is – like a fire alarm. Hoping I won't have to use those skills! One more lesson next week, and I will be signed off, which means that Max and I will be able to wander across to the playroom at will, without a constant nurse escort. However, Max will still require two nurses when he leaves the ward because he is on Milrinone and Dobutamine. Paul will get his training next week too.

Later on Saturday, the lovely Norma came to visit and brought Max some Domino's chicken wings and heart-shaped watermelon slices! He ate them all, so his appetite seems better. Norma and I then went to dinner at my favourite table at The Victory. Fab!

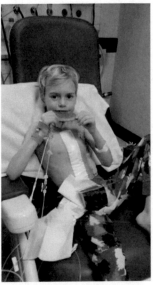

Max enjoying watermelon in intensive care
Photo Credit: Emma Johnson

"A really positive post. Lovely when things are going so well xx, Liz C."

"Emma, that all sounds like a good week for you. When you said six months, I was taken aback. Where does the time go? Max is so inspiring and you and Paul give us so much…thank you. Love to Harry, Paul, you and the incredible Max. xxx Malcolm."

"Glad to hear another positive week. Keep up the good work, Max and team. We remember you in our prayers every night and send lots of love and big smiles from Gary too x. Liz."

It was always going to be a real challenge to get Max to put weight on, even though we were ostensibly only seeking to replace the weight he'd lost since falling ill. End stage heart failure wreaks havoc on all of your organs – they are not getting the blood they need – but the tummy really lets you know about it. Max would quite regularly suffer with bouts of sickness and tummy ache, which made his norovirus and clostridium difficile, a gut infection, an even crueller blow. Over the months of his stay in hospital, a number of different tactics were deployed to give him the calories he needed.

Interestingly, there were a couple of gastronomic delights that Max always managed to have an appetite for; McDonald's fries (as mentioned) and Domino's chicken wings – the latter being quite a costly option over time! Never mind, such was the desperation of the situation that the funds were made available (thank you Barclaycard) so that Max could eat his herb coated delights and be washed and ready for bed by handover time at 8 o'clock in the evening. Along with smoked salmon and watermelon, the costs soon mounted.

Sadly, this was not enough, so other weight gain strategies were required. Max, who was given a choice between apple or banana, was put onto a calorie-heavy fruit drink, and he was required to consume some 600ml per day. A significant inroad into his total daily fluid allowance. It was, in fairness to Max, like drinking syrup and offered little by way of desirable flavour or texture. To his apple juice, or any other drink, we also had to add a colourless and flavourless powder, which further boosted the calorific content. Colourless and flavourless, eh? Maybe to an elderly patient with a diminished awareness of skulduggery, but Max became a dab hand at identifying when we were trying to feed him these extra calories. Our attempted subterfuge exposed, he would become quite cross if his beloved cold milk had been tampered with, and on many occasions, we had to concede defeat and present him with a fresh, unadulterated replacement.

There is a very serious point to this. As I have alluded before, being at an optimum weight is really important before transplant. It was said – many times – that the outcome would be much better if Max had more weight on him. It's just that convincing a little boy with a poorly, achy tummy and zero appetite that he really does need to drink this heavy, sticky apple drink, would be a hard sell even for Del Boy. Moreover, there was the hovering spectre of a feeding tube being required and the efforts to get Max to drink these juices and eat his McDonald's were all to convince the dieticians that he did not need to have the tube. When all is said and done, you will do what you need to do in the best interests of your child, but Max had been so traumatised when the first tube was fitted in late January, that the prospect of a second tube being mandated was a constant worry. Indeed, the scars from the experience inflicted during the fitting of that first tube had become seared into Max's consciousness; the feeding tube really was his nemesis.

Regrettably, Max's food intake was still insufficient. On several occasions, the lead dietician travelled to see Max from the nearby Royal Victoria Infirmary to assess his case. During every visit, real concerns were expressed about Max's long-term prospects if he did not manage to gain weight. As parents, we felt hugely responsible for this, but utterly helpless and near powerless to influence things, no matter how hard we tried. It was exhausting. Everything was being done to prevent the need for a new feeding tube, but options were limited, so the dark, menacing and ever elongating shadow of a second tube continued to encroach.

We had developed a new system of Cockney Rhyming Slang for the various ports, drips and drains entering Max's body. We had time on our hands! Let me explain; his Hickman line, through which he received his IV drugs and from which his bloods were taken, was now called his 'Alan Rickman'…Alan Rickman – Hickman. His Milrinone – that vital life-sustaining drug with which I had a real love hate relationship was called 'Moan and Groan'…Moan and Groan – Milrinone. Finally came the TPN (Total Parenteral Nutrition), and this was linked with Max's need to gain weight. The TPN, in effect, put food directly into his blood stream. As you may surmise from this route one approach, the TPN, or 'Mother Hen', was not ideal; additional pressure on Max's liver and a significantly raised risk of infection. Both risks were a concern, but the latter came with an additional menace. If Max picked up an infection, there would be a real chance that he would have to come off the urgent transplant list and that could have, quite literally, fatal consequences for him.

We persevered with the Mother Hen for a few short weeks – on top of the risks, it had to be specially prepared and started at a certain time during the evening…and the TPN machine was quite temperamental and given to bouts of hissy fitting. So, we can conclude that there was not much to recommend Mother Hen in Max's case. That said, it would be remiss not to acknowledge that for some, it is a lifesaver. We had run out of options. With nervousness and perhaps a sense of inevitability, the decision was made to fit another feeding tube. Max was only getting half of what he needed from the Mother Hen, and it wasn't really delivering gains, just an unsatisfactory status quo. In conjunction with Kathryn and Sue of the psychology team and with the full backing of the dieticians, an approach was decided upon to break the news to Max.

More than anything that happened to him, Max's biggest fear was the NGT. It was agreed that it would be put in place under general anaesthetic – not the norm, especially due to his very weak heart – but allowances were being made for Max. This was another example of how the team did everything they could to do the right thing by Max. It was a true and kind concession to his thoughts, feelings and fears in deciding his treatment and how best to administer it.

Sue and Kathryn thought that the news should be broken to Max by Dr Reinhardt. They believed that if he saw that the instruction was coming from the top and from someone not involved with him on a day-to-day basis, the message would at least hit home as both serious and non-negotiable. It did. We sat in the newly decorated adolescent room, this time on the red vinyl seats, and Dr Reinhardt broke the news to Max. I felt such a traitor – I had told Max that we needed to speak with Dr Reinhardt and he thought that he may be going home – I said that this was not the case (heart-breaking nonetheless), but that we needed to have a chat with her. I believe that Max suspected the reason, but he kept his powder dry.

As Dr Reinhardt spoke with Max, he slumped to the floor and his eyes filled with tears – he pleaded with me; "I don't want it. Please, Dad, I don't want a feeding tube!" As he spoke, he banged his head hard against the arm of the chair. By virtue of the fact that his blood was already thinned with Warfarin due to the LVAD pump, I gently restrained him; a bleed on the brain could sign, seal and deliver his fate. We all tried to calm him – it was in his best interests

– but there was no consoling him. Dr Reinhardt, her role played as requested, left the room and so did the play specialist, Karen, so that I could talk with Max. He sat on my knee, the tears flowing down his cheeks. "Today is the day I give up, Dad, I've had enough!" His words cut me to my core and I remembered the night standing outside the Indian restaurant in Winsford, when Max was told of the possible need for a new heart. I couldn't help it – I started to cry. I was shattered. Max had come this far in no small part due to his resilience, his fight, his good humour – his sheer determination – but here he genuinely seemed to be saying it had gone. Emma had seen the impact of the first feeding tube; this time, we knew where we were heading.

Max turned and looked at me and saw the tears flowing down my cheeks. "Please don't give up, Max, I don't want to lose you…" Max fixed his gaze on me and with his right hand, he gently wiped the tears from my cheek.

Through his own tears, he said, "Don't cry, Dad…I don't like seeing you cry." I told him I was sorry and then there was a moment where we both just held one another and I gently kissed the top of his head.

Max broke the silence. "Okay, Dad, I'll have the tube…in fact, I'll probably look forward for it."

Max has a sweet way of saying 'for it' instead of 'to it'. I wept again, but this time, my tears were tears of relative happiness and wonder, that yet again, this priceless little boy had rallied. I wrapped my arms around him and hugged him as tightly as I dared. *You little fighter,* I thought. Karen came back in and we made our way out into the corridor, where we were joined by Max's nurse and the sister. As Max walked on ahead, the sister looked at me. With an unspoken comprehension of my emotional exhaustion, she rubbed my arm and said, "Well done." I was spent and I knew that the road ahead would still be rocky, but the decision we had made felt like the right one, and in time, it proved to be so.

The procedure was scheduled for the following day. Max remained positive for the rest of the afternoon, evening and following morning, but I sensed that his joie de vivre was more for my benefit than heartfelt. As the 'premeds' were administered, Max had the now customary mood swings and I again could not help feeling that they were the inner, unsuppressed anxieties being given voice. The whole thing was over in thirty minutes, but as we collected Max from the recovery room, we could again see – as with the first tube – that something had been extinguished. He was taken downstairs and lay in his bed, not moving and not talking, just looking out at the 'Tree of Life'.

It was like this for the best part of a week. Max's customary sense of humour had gone, and he communicated by jutting his jaw forwards, which in turn gave him a difficult to understand, and unfortunately, quite comical nasal sound to his speech. Max was not in on the joke – and who could blame him – he was fed up. With almost biblical timing, on the seventh day, things started to look up. Max had noticed for himself that he was slowly gaining weight with the feeding tube, and although it had made him sick a couple of times, he was getting used to the creamy liquid it delivered every night; this time into his tummy and via nature's approved route of the gut, rather than straight into the blood stream. Another boon for Max was that he was feeling a bit stronger and was about to enjoy his longest, sustained period of relative, clinical stability. His need for a new heart retained its urgency, but hopefully, this improved weight, strength and wellbeing would put Max in the box seat ahead of his little gift arriving.

DIARY OF A HEART MUM: Twenty-Second Weekly Update – Sunday. 18 June, 2017.

A week 'difficile': 'Odds and Gods'

Well! A terrible week! On Monday, the head honcho, Dr Reinhardt, broke the news to Max that the following day, he would be having a feeding tube. Despite reassurances that this was not a 'punishment' and that his weight loss was not Max's fault, he reacted very badly and Paul said that he was extremely angry and upset! With the help of the team, by the evening, Max had accepted his fate, and when I spoke to Max on Monday night, he told me that he felt "nervous, but happy", but his voice was shaky.

On Tuesday morning, Max was taken up to intensive care for a general anaesthetic to fit the tube. They gave him some 'funny' medicine, to make him relaxed and Paul said that Max was singing Ed Sheeran's 'Shape of You' in a 'drunkard' fashion, and he told the play specialist that she had 'a big nose, but lovely white teeth!' He denied being Max Johnson, saying, "I'm not Max! Max is at home!" and that his birth date was '3rd Jan 23'! I sweated it out at work waiting for the call that Max was safely through the procedure.

Max was really depressed and sad waking up to the feeding tube. I arrived on Wednesday afternoon, and he was in a terrible state – gagging, quiet, sad and staring out of the window, forlorn. He can't speak well with the feeding tube and juts his bottom jaw forward to try and relieve the feeling in his throat. All day Thursday, poor Max was gagging and retching constantly due to the tube. Lots of cuddling, soothing and stroking!

On Friday morning, Max seemed to improve and was gagging less. He even started to write a list of places he wants to go to when he is better. However, he had also been suffering from terrible diarrhoea since Tuesday, so a sample had been sent off. I can't help wondering whether the 'Odds and Gods' are against me, because on Friday afternoon, precisely 30 minutes after my final HeartWare Training session in which I was officially 'signed off' to travel around the ward and playroom with Max independently, the doctors told me that the sample results showed that Max had a gut infection called 'Chlostridium Difficile'. He and the family would need to stay in his bed space and not mix with any other patients and families, to prevent infection spread! They even put 'infection tape' around his bed space, as if it was a crime scene! You couldn't write it!

On Friday evening though, the staff allowed the lovely Andrea (Harry's best friend from primary school, Will's Mum) to visit Max, as long as there was plenty of handwashing. Max was very subdued, but I really think he was pleased to see Andrea, who was so good with him. She brought him some fantastic books to read. Andrea and I went for tea at my usual table at The Victory and had a lovely chat! Thank you, Andrea!

By Saturday morning, Max looked terrible; he was obviously dehydrated due to the runs and his face and eyes looked hollow. He had suffered a number of disturbed nights with retching/sickness and diarrhoea, so was completely exhausted. The doctor decided he needed Dioralyte to rehydrate him and started him on antibiotics to kill the 'c-difficile' bug. Paul and Harry had arrived late Friday night and they were able to cheer Max up, and throughout Saturday, Max started to improve, although fragile.

By Sunday morning, the playroom was cleared to allow Max and the family out into the Playroom Garden. Max watered the sunflowers that he had planted and watered us too, which he took great delight in! He played ball with Harry and seemed a lot better, both physically and spiritually. The antibiotics seem to be working and at least he's not allergic to this lot!

I took Harry and Paul to The Victory for Sunday lunch for Father's Day, but couldn't help feeling sad with 'the empty chair'. It reminded me of the song from 'Les Mis' – 'Empty chairs at empty tables'. Paul is an amazing husband and father and I don't know how our family would have coped all this time without him! Harry and I arrived back in Cheshire on Sunday evening, ready for school and work on Monday! Very tired! So, a bad week, ending cautiously optimistic!

"Oh, Emma. I'm always thinking of you all, and I count my blessings when I tuck my two into bed. Sending all of our love and hugs xx, Fiona."

"Always thinking about you and how exhausted you must be. Max is lucky in one thing – his parents and their devotion and steadfastness. Hope this nightmare does not last much longer, and that he is soon on the road to recovery xx, Liz C."

"You have all had a very bad time and we're so sorry. There is only one way though now and that's up! The strength that you all have will hopefully make the climb easier and let's hope the view from the top will be better. Lots of love to Harry, Paul, yourself and brave Max. xxx Malcolm."

"Hey – another tough week – but look – you're all coming through it – fantastic! Well done. Keep fighting and keep positive – even if all you feel you can do is to not be negative – it's a great place to start at those moments when you feel 'low'. You make a strong unit – the four of you – long may it continue that way. We're all with you in spirit – willing you on and sending good vibes! I can hear Dad (Albert) saying, 'He who fights and runs away, lives to fight another day!' I think it's so. Love and hugs, Suzanne xxxx."

"Emma, you've just made me cry with the news of what a difficult week you have all had (especially Max). I hope the worst is over for Max with the feeding tube and that he grows more used to it as the days go by with less gagging. I can't imagine it is very pleasant! Tell him that I am thinking about him and rooting for him and that he must stay strong. The children and staff loved the card he sent from 'The Toon', which I read out in assembly on Friday. You are right – Paul is amazing, as you all are, for staying so strong and being there for each other. All my love, thoughts and best wishes, Alex XX."

'*What a difference a week makes!*' What a turnaround! Max has had a much better week and he seems to have got used to his feeding tube. The extra '*energy*' he is getting from the '*NG*' tube is palpable! He even has an appetite, and so is eating a bit more. He is back to his impish self, which is a joy to behold after last week's slide!

In terms of the '*C-difficile*' bug, Max was given the all clear on Friday, and so we had to go through another '*bed space*' deep clean. This included me washing all his clothes, cuddly toys, duvet, everything...in the Scott House laundry! Every item belonging to Max had to be cleaned with desanitiser chemical! Took ages! It frustrates me that not every parent washes their hands when they enter the ward. I believe this leaves children like Max vulnerable to bugs! Have had a diplomatic word with the sister about educating people about the importance of handwashing and I think she will send out a general letter and improve signage. I must admit, in the early months, I thought washing my hands with the gel was sufficient, until I discovered that bugs like '*Chlostridium Difficile*' can survive gel, but not handwashing. This kind of information should be shared with all parents, as how are we to know?

Max excelled himself with his sense of humour this week and I think he is developing my own liking for plays on words. We were in the shop on a wheelchair walk and Max noticed a customer grappling with the coffee machine, which had a small sign saying '*Out of Order*'. Max explained to the man that the machine was broken and the man said thank you and had a little grumble. Max replied with, "I know...It's WELL out of order!" – A young man after my own heart! Not literally! Although, if I could swap, I would! Also, this week, a nurse said to Max: "You have four lovely nurses looking after you..."

Max replied: "All my dreams have come true!" Gotta love him!

On Saturday, I finally got to explore the playroom/playroom garden and parents' room, with just Max and no nurse escort. What bliss! Not being listened to and watched constantly, which is very exhausting! FREEDOM! However, I am slave to his drip stand, as I follow him around making sure his wires don't tug!

We have had a lovely response to the call for raffle prizes in aid of The Sick Children's Trust at Neil's garden party. Bose have sent a Soundlink Mini 11 Speaker, Manchester United have sent a load of goodies, thanks to Max's not-so-evil Godmother, Helen, and also a signed shirt, thanks to Neil. Newcastle United are donating a signed ball (again…thank you, Auntie Helen!). To top it all, David Walliams replied to my letter. He wrote a lovely bespoke letter to Paul and me, and sent two signed copies of his new book, one for the raffle and one for Max (he included signed photographs). I am even more of a fan now! He must get loads of post, so was very touched.

Another boost – our vicar, Chris, wrote a beautiful prayer for our family, which he read on Tuesday evening at the 'Lost in Translation' evening that I agreed to do. This involved talking about The Sick Children's Trust (Chris showed a film of Neil and Harry training for their run next Saturday). Then, after the tea break, Chris interviewed me about miscommunication that can occur between differences in culture (Japanese and British). We finished the night with a drink in the Old Star with Chris and his lovely family! The evening raised £250 towards The Sick Children's Trust!

Finally, look out for Max's story in the Mirror newspaper tomorrow (Monday, 26 June). The Sick Children's Trust has a partnership with the Mirror, as the newspaper is running a campaign about organ donation and also supports the charity. Fingers crossed it appears and raises awareness on a national level.

Well, that's all, folks! Thank you for all your love and support. Love, Em X.

"What a fantastic update, Emma. So glad the feeding tube is not troubling Max and his appetite and sense of humour have returned. Lovely to read about the amazing response to the raffle, the lovely church event and the letter from David Walliams. Love, Gill."

"You all continue to amaze me as you journey through the ups and downs. Fingers crossed for more ups like this. Love to all, Nic xx."

"Emma, I'm so thrilled to read such a lovely positive message – you, Paul, Harry and of course Max are all my heroes and whether times are tough or more positive, you still keep your focus, pull together and stay strong in your love for each other. I've got some goodies for Max as well as some watermelon ice cubes so will pop over. Do you fancy a bite out this weekend, or maybe an in-ward picnic again with Max? Much love, Norma xxx."

"Sounds like you've had a much better week, Emma. That is great to hear as I was really worrying about Max after your last update. I'm up to £900 now on the JustGiving page and I'm going to go for a new target of £2,000 between now and my next race in September. All our love, thoughts and prayers, Alex X."

Chapter 9

It was not an easy decision to get involved in the Mirror campaign to Change the Law for Life. It was even harder choosing the appropriate photograph of Max that we knew would have the possibility of featuring on the front page of the Mirror. We poured over several photographs, but there was one that stood out. It was a harrowing photograph of Max which captured the juxtaposition of Max's broken, failing and underweight body against the expression and spirit of human hope and optimism in fighting adversity, with that half-smile and begging eyes. If any image was going to have a significant impact, this was the one.

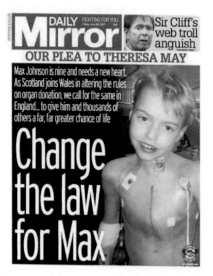

Max's first appearance on the front cover of the Mirror
Photo Credit: Emma Johnson/Mirror Newspaper Group

Emma remembers sharing the photograph with her friends and family on Facebook saying, "Max wanted me to post this photograph. He is feeling a bit sad and fragile today. His Hickman line that feeds the Milrinone to his heart blocked up on Monday, and yesterday he had a general anaesthetic to put in a new Hickman Line. He is in some discomfort and distress…but even in difficult spells, he always says please and thank you. Please think of him tonight. Love, Em x."

The image really hammered home to our friends and family just how poorly our son had become and there were tears shed that evening, I know.

Before we sent the photo through to Jeremy Armstrong at the Mirror Newspaper, we asked ourselves why we were agreeing to allow Max to be in the public eye. There were two main reasons. We agreed that the law should change, so that members of the public would have the choice of 'opting out' as well as 'opting in' to organ donation. If you didn't 'opt in' or 'opt out', then organ donation consent would be 'deemed'. We felt that a law change could raise awareness, increase the number of 'known decisions', thus increasing the consent rate and reducing the wait for anybody of any age needing an organ transplant. We also understood that any law change would result in a 'soft opt out' system, meaning that the family would still have the final say. What clinched the decision? Max also gave his blessing for the sharing of this, oh so personal, photograph. He understood that it could help him and help others also.

We knew what it felt like to have a loved one 'languishing', 'deteriorating' on 'death row'. It was like torture, purgatory, highly emotional and both physically and mentally draining. If there was anything we could do to reduce this stress for others, then we were prepared to chip in. The other big reason was a selfish one. We felt that sharing Max's story might just strike a chord with a bereaved family and result in consent to organ donation, which might not otherwise be forthcoming. In other words, it might just result in Max getting that precious gift. We understood the power of the media and we would do anything, if there was the slightest chance that Max would be saved. We also felt that if we didn't share Max's story and if Max didn't make it in time for a new heart, that we would always regret not getting behind the campaign and potentially making a difference.

When Emma first met with Jeremy Armstrong to be interviewed face to face following a phone chat, she was at a very low ebb and finding it incredibly hard to stay positive. She felt bedraggled, exhausted and was at a point where she was just too distraught to worry about how she looked. However, her feeling unkempt was magnified when she first met the well-groomed and crisp-suited reporter. *Oh Lord! I should have made a bit of an effort! What a contrast!* she thought. She was very nervous and had no idea what to expect. She was anxious that words would be twisted or that accuracy might be compromised in favour of sensationalism. She soon felt at ease and was relieved that Jeremy was blessed with empathy and understanding, as she really didn't know what your typical tabloid reporter would be like. That empathy and understanding was rooted in tragic personal experience; he had lost his 35-year-old best friend to undiagnosed cardiomyopathy some years back. There was a genuine interest in Max's story and the illness that had befallen him. This clearly wasn't just about selling newspapers; there was a very noble cause to fight. We were very impressed that Jeremy always sent us his articles in draft to check before they were published, which helped to build a feeling of trust and assurance. Little did we realise how Max's story and the Mirror campaign to Change the Law for Life would snowball and that Max would appear on the front page of the Mirror no fewer than fifteen times over the coming months and into 2018.

Jeremy and Max also became good buddies. Jeremy even took part in the Great North Run in 2017 in honour of Max's story and in memory of his best friend, Dave. He gave his medal to Max – a lovely gesture – "You've got more chance of becoming President of the US than getting one of these, Dad," said Harry. *Thanks, Son.*

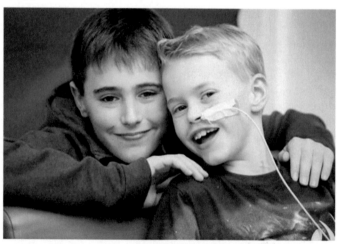

Max and Harry
Photo Credit: Andy Commins/Mirror Newspaper Group

The headlines that ran whilst Max was still ill and waiting for his heart were quite harrowing. The first article with 'that' picture was published on 26 June 2017, with the headline:

'CHANGE THE LAW FOR MAX – Max Johnson is 9 and needs a new heart. As Scotland joins Wales in altering the rules on organ donation, we call for the same in England to give him and thousands of others a far, far greater chance of life.'

Other articles followed with similar themes:

'"We want England as well": Desperate Mum calls for change in organ donation laws before time runs out for her critically ill son.'

But then the mood changed to one of optimism, as the government started to listen and respond:

'Hope for critically ill Max, 9, as Theresa May promises, "We are looking at organ donation law".'

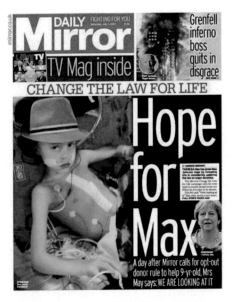

Front page of the Mirror 'Hope for Max'
Photo Credit: Emma Johnson/Mirror Newspaper Group

The Mirror continued to run articles about Max, to put pressure on the government, such as:

'The tiny metal pump weighing just 160g that is keeping Max Johnson alive as he awaits new heart.'

'"Please save my life, Prime Minister": Heart transplant boy Max Johnson in plea to change donor law.'

By now, the Mirror had also set up a public petition to collect signatures of those that agreed that such a law change was overdue.

'Pressure mounts on Theresa May to change organ donor laws as Mirror appeal hits 10,000 supporters.'

'Little Max's fight for a new heart reaches Parliament as his parents push to change organ donor law.'

We were both quite anxious about how the hospital staff would view Max's involvement in the Mirror's crusade. As the articles gathered pace and Max featured more and more as the 'Poster Boy' of the Change the Law for Life campaign, we felt that support from the hospital team, also started to gain traction.

DIARY OF A HEART MUM: Twenty-Fourth Weekly Update – Sunday, 2 July 2017.

Max has had another good week and his weight is gaining. He weighed 23 kg this morning, so much improved and the feeding tube is doing its job.

Max was the DJ at another patient's birthday party on Friday. A lovely seven-year-old girl who is waiting for her second heart transplant, as the first one didn't work out. Max loved stopping the music for 'Pass the Parcel' and he didn't seem to mind that he was missing out on opening the parcel. There was a fantastic magician/comedian at the party and it was lovely seeing all the children from the ward, forgetting their woes and giggling away.

It was a busy week in terms of the media. The Sick Children's Trust Press Office had contacted us about sharing our story to help with their fundraising. We have been staying at Scott House free of charge all year, so we felt the need to try and help. The Press Office sent the press release to the Mirror newspaper, who seemed very keen on running the story and reigniting their campaign to 'Change the Law for Life'. Max was featured three times this week, Monday, Friday and Saturday, and the campaign has really gained momentum. On Monday, there was an uplift of 1000 extra people registering for organ donation and the petition to change the law rose to nearly 6000 in two days!

We have had massive support for our decision to share the story (which wasn't an easy decision!), but who knows, Max may get the 'gift of life' that he needs through raising awareness. Hey, if I can sell protein powder in Japan, I might as well use my marketing skills to try and get my son a heart! But on a serious note, if this issue is in people's consciousness and if something dreadful happened to a family member, the next of kin may be slightly more inclined to say 'yes' to agreeing for their loved one to donate organs, rather than saying 'no'. The people who I have come into contact with, who have made this difficult decision, consistently say what comfort it brings to know that their loved ones have saved others. Most people don't know that one organ donor can save or transform up to nine lives. What an incredible gift and a beautiful legacy!

Max has discovered the small bicycle in the playroom garden! He loves riding it round and round, but I have to scurry behind with his drip stand so that his wires don't pull! Nightmare, but at least he is having fun! He is really enjoying having his friend, Dylan, in the next bed.

Saturday was a busy day for all the family. Harry, Neil and the lovely Jennifer, succeeded in completing their 5K run in Chester. Paul, Auntie Lottie, Sammy, Max, William, Chris, Avril and Jill were there to cheer them on. They have smashed their target for The Sick Children's Trust of £2000 and the pot stands at £2077 and that's without the church event donations of £250 and without the raffle at Neil's garden party.

On the other side of the country, Max was visited by Uncle Roger, James, Edward and William. They played together so nicely in the playroom garden and Max was in his element! Norma arrived with watermelon ice cubes and space stickers for Max and we then retired to The Victory for food and LARGE gin and tonics! Lovely! Feeling positive!

"Wow, Em! What a fab positive week! So happy for you all. Well done to Harry, Neil and Jennifer too – superb performance! Thrilled too about the fact that so many people are getting involved in raising awareness! Long may it continue! Much love from us all xx, Janis."

"So wonderful to see Max looking so well and happy and to have a good old splurge with you on Saturday night – just the job! Much love to you all and look forward to seeing Paul this week x, Norma."

"Thank you, Emma, for making us feel both relieved and better after a really good week. It sounds like Max is tackling new ventures that help him and the gin and tonic helps you along too! Love to Paul, Harry, you and wonderful Max xxxx. Malcolm."

"Wonderful update, Emma! So glad you have all had another positive week and long may it continue. Xx Elaine."

DIARY OF A HEART MUM: Twenty-Fifth Weekly Update – Sunday, 9 July 2017.

Another positive week and Max continues to gain weight with the help of the feeding tube.

I personally haven't been to Newcastle this week, but Paul has been there doing a sterling job and Max is stable, although he does tire easily. He can get lively and forgets that his heart has limits and will then need to rest in bed and recover.

Max is now the official 'poster boy' of the 'Change the Law for Life campaign' and as I write this, 8749 have signed the petition. In the meantime though, more and more people are signing the Organ Donor Register.

We feel very supported by the Freeman Hospital, with Mr Hasan, the paediatric heart surgeon giving quotes to the Mirror too, in support of a law change.

One of the doctors said to Max: "So, Max, you are a celebrity now!"

To which Max replied, "I know! Get me out of here!"

I met with Harry's counsellor and form tutor on Thursday and they gave some very good advice about helping Harry over the summer. Despite being given exemption from the first year exams, he managed to get a fantastic report and even got a MERIT badge from his form teacher, which he will wear on his blazer from September. Really proud of him, as he has been having a tough time with all the upheaval!

Harry and I went to see Mum, Dad and Marcus on Friday, and Harry stayed there whilst I went for my heart check at the Heart Centre in Manchester. This is in case the cause of Max's illness is genetic. Paul is just waiting for his appointment letter. I have the all-clear (as does Harry).

Returned to have tea with Mum and Dad and then Harry and I set off for a mini-break in Cumbria near Lake Derwent. We had a lovely day on Saturday, walking and a boat trip. We stayed in a little B&B in a farmhouse at the top of the hills near Ashness Bridge. It was nice and old-fashioned, and we got two delicious breakfasts. On Sunday morning, we met Neil, Jennifer and Jennifer's two children, Mabel and Seb, on the banks of Lake Derwent. Neil succeeded in completing the open water swim for The Sick Children's Trust. Had a lovely lunch in Keswick to celebrate Neil's achievement and headed back to Cheshire.

Spoke with Paul and all fine with Max. Max was visited by Norma on Saturday and by Gramps on Sunday.

Crisis at The Victory: one chef down and an hour delay on food! How will I cope when I return to Newcastle on Wednesday night!

P.S: Harry and I have been invited by MP Dan Jarvis and the Mirror to attend Prime Minister's question time on Wednesday, as they are discussing the 'opt out' law. The Mirror is organising our train tickets and also a pass to go on a tour of The House of Commons. Harry has never even been to London, let alone PMQ!

Harry and I have discussed this and agree that it is sensible to try and channel our energy into positive, productive activities that might just help Max, rather than negative thoughts and feelings! (Easier said than done!)

I have a feeling Max's heart will come over the summer!

"I also have a good feeling that Max's new heart will come over the summer, Emma; it is strange but I have thought this for a long time, so I'm willing this to come true with my whole being. It's great that you have had such a positive week and that Max is stable and doing well. See you soon when I come up to Geordie land again! Love, Alex."

"So glad that this week was so positive, Em, and delighted that the Mirror campaign is doing so much to highlight the issue of organ donation! Glad too that you enjoyed your much-needed break! Much love to all xx, Janis."

"So glad that you had a break and such a lovely time with Harry. You really needed the mini holiday. Delighted to hear Dan Jarvis this morning. Not only mentioning Max, but also you and Harry, *and said you were in the gallery! Hope that this week is as positive as last week was! x Liz C."*

"It's great to have the distraction of the Mirror campaign, but also a huge extra burden to take on. Well done for embracing this opportunity in such a positive way. Feel free to plan some time for Harry to come over with us. We'd love to go up to Delamere again sometime over the holidays; he is always more than welcome to come for a stay for a few days. We would love to help pour some cooling water on those overheating cores and avoid a meltdown! I'm so pleased you got a chance to have a break for a while in the Lakes. Will be chortling about Max's, 'I'm a celebrity, get me out of here' joke for a while. Love, Nic xx."

When Dan Jarvis MP invited Emma and Harry to attend Prime Minister's question time in July, where he was seeking to raise a question about changing the organ donation law, it was a no-brainer that they should attend. It also allowed Harry to feel that he was contributing and gave him a positive focus, as he had been struggling to cope with Max's ordeal and having such a fragmented family. Emma and Harry were well looked after in London and they were shown around the Palace of Westminster. They were ushered to a seat in the gallery, where they could see Dan Jarvis MP, who stood up and said:

"Little Max Johnson is nine. He is in hospital, and he is urgently waiting for a heart transplant. His Mum, Emma, and his brother, Harry, join us today to support Max, but also the thousands of people around the country who need an organ transplant. We can do more to help them. Wales has already moved to the 'opt out' system, and Scotland plans to do the same. Does the First Secretary agree with me that, in England, we should change the law to one of presumed consent for organ donation, to give Max and all those other people the best chance of life?"

The response from PM Theresa May's deputy, Damian Green MP, was:

"I am sure that the thoughts of members across the House are with Max and his family at this incredibly difficult time. I agree with the hon. Gentleman that organ donation is clearly a hugely important part of our system, and I am pleased that there are now more than 23 million people on the Organ Donor Register. Over the past year, we saw the highest ever donor and transplant rates in the UK, but of course, there is more that can be done. As the hon Gentleman says, the law is different in other territories inside the

UK, and the Department of Health is looking at the impact of those changes to see if they can give rise to further improvements in the number of available organs."

Emma described the experience as strangely surreal. It was difficult to comprehend that the little boy being referred to was her little boy. Emma and Harry were encouraged by the government's response that seemed to bode well for considered reflection. Despite the positives of the trip, Emma felt completely drained on the journey home after being 'on show'. It took a great deal of courage, but the issues were so important. She didn't want any personal, social fear to get in the way of possible progress. We had agreed to support the Mirror's crusade and we were in for a penny, in for a pound.

Shortly afterwards, Geoffrey Robinson presented the first reading of the 'Organ Donation Deemed Consent Bill', with a date set for 23 February 2018 for the second reading of the bill. One small step closer to law change!

DIARY OF A HEART MUM: Twenty-Sixth Weekly Update – Sunday, 16 July 2017.

Max has had another brilliant week. In fact, I think this is the most stable that he has been. There is no change in the function of Max's heart, but he continues to gain weight and the feeding tube is definitely giving him balanced nutrition, which is giving him more energy.

On Monday, had a lovely visit from Max's Godmother, Helen, who has managed to secure some amazing raffle prizes for the raffle for The Sick Children's Trust. Thank you, Helen!

Worked Monday and Tuesday – very busy and managing to contribute, despite everything!

The Mirror campaign to 'Change the Law for Life' went up a gear and Harry and I travelled to London on the train, whilst Paul looked after Max. We watched Dan Jarvis, MP for Barnsley, present a question about Max and the organ donation law from up in the gallery. Very bizarre and a really fascinating insight. Harry and I got to see the procession of the Speaker of the House carrying the gold mace and we saw the spot where Winston Churchill lay in state. We got to London in good time, so we got off at Green Park and I showed Harry where I used to work at The Embassy of Japan, then went past Buckingham Palace and through St James Park to Westminster. Dan Jarvis, his aides and the Mirror staff made us feel so welcome and greeted us with respect and kindness. Really bowled over!

We made our way back to Crewe on the train. Got home, tidied up, packed and then I set off for Newcastle. Met Paul at Wetherby Services! What a guy! Got to Newcastle at midnight as the A1 was closed!

On Thursday, I had coffee at the hospital with Jeremy Armstrong from the Mirror, who explained more about the goal of the campaign and thanked us for our help. Very humbling to be involved and helps us all on a psychological level to channel some energy in such a positive and productive way! Lots of hospital staff approaching me to say that they think the Mirror campaign is fantastic and that, even if the change in law isn't voted in, the awareness raising and debating around the topic can only be a good thing! We continue to be grateful for and hugely impressed with the outstanding work and attitude of the staff that we come into contact with!

The Victory is better and back to normal service. So, Norma and I celebrated with a meal there. She brought Max some watermelon and a protective eagle to hang over Max's bed. The landlady of The Victory gave us a complimentary meal and two bottles of wine for The Sick Children's Trust raffle. Just lovely!

I have started putting one hour aside every day for a power walk down through Freeman Park, along the river in Jesmond Dene, past the waterfalls and down to the Petting Zoo. Then back up the hill and round to the hospital. It is always poignant when I see animals, as I know how much Max would love them. Anyway, at least I am trying to do some exercise and shift some of the weight I have put on.

Another child, an eight-year-old, has got their heart transplant and overtaken Max. Fantastic news for that family, but poor Max, why is it always him who is left waiting!

"Delighted that the week has been a positive one. Thinking of you every day and praying that life is onwards and upwards for you xxxxxxx, Steve."

"Lovely post. So much to take in still. Much love to all, Nic xx."

"Good to hear that Max has had a good week. Good lad. We have loved reading all the articles in the papers. You are all so caring to cope with this. Today, I send you love from sunny France. Cahors is as lovely as ever, and I am trying out the Cahors wine with great enthusiasm. Love to Paul, Harry, great Max and to you, Emma. Malcolm."

"Great news, Emma, keep hanging in there – it sounds like it has been a very positive week. The trip down to London sounds very exciting! Alex X."

DIARY OF A HEART MUM: Twenty-Sixth Weekly Update – Sunday, 16 July 2017.

NONE

DIARY OF A HEART MUM: Twenty-Seventh Weekly Update – Sunday, 23 July 2017.

Max has had another good week, despite a driveline infection, making the port swollen, red and weepy. However, this was blitzed with 48 hours IV antibiotics (not the same family as the ones he was allergic to!) followed by oral antibiotics. So, fine, and Max's weight has stabilised at about 23.7 kg. This is ideal for accepting a new heart. Max is still pranking. He put a McDonald's chip on his shoulder and loved saying to everyone "I've got a chip on my shoulder" because "I'm a chip off the old block".

I came home on Monday, and for the first time, Harry, Paul and I had an evening together in Cheshire and we went to the newly refurbed Vale Royal Abbey Arms for tea. It was lovely! Watched the rabbits out on the grassy bank and thought of Max who used to love chasing them! Can't wait to bring him back when better.

We all met Auntie Charlotte (Harry's Godmother) at St Luke's Coffee Shop on Delamere Street. It was lovely to see her twin boys, Max and Will. They are really growing up and so polite and well behaved.

Paul travelled off to Newcastle straight after and I have booked the week off work (and next week). Harry enjoyed a relaxing week without the pressures of school.

Harry took me to Whitegate Way on Wednesday. He rolled along on his Swegway and he got me jogging. So unfit! Trying to shift some weight but very difficult. Managed two Zumba sessions too; one with Helena from St Chad's Church and one at The Winsford Lifestyle Centre.

On Wednesday morning, I also met with my friend, Liz, in the St Luke's Coffee Shop, so that was lovely. I have known Liz for many years and she is a true friend.

The Mirror campaign went up a gear and the MP, Geoffrey Robinson, presented the first reading for the 'Organ Donation Deemed Consent Bill' (affectionately dubbed 'Max's Law'). The second reading will be 23 February 2018 when there will be a big debate and then I think MPs vote. So, the Mirror campaign has definitely helped to push this through. On Monday, the reporter at the Mirror, Jeremy, will be writing a piece about what it is like waiting for an organ, so a different angle, but one that could help people understand how awful the wait is and that the change of law could help to reduce the time and suffering spent waiting. The petition to change the law is now over 10,000.

Harry and I travelled back to Cheshire and we ended up listening to Gardener's Question time on BBC Radio 4 and were laughing about the fact that how luxurious a life would be if all you had to worry about were a collapsing courgette, wilting wisteria and cat poo in your garden!

Neil and Jennifer hosted their annual Garden Party on Saturday and The Sick Children's Trust raffle raised over £700. Max drew the winning tickets through a live video link from the playroom in Newcastle with Chris, the vicar, orchestrating and announcing the prizes and winning tickets back in Cheshire.

It was so touching and lovely to see the winners thrilled with their prizes as we had worked so hard to gather them from companies/individuals. The party was such fun, with a live artist and it was nice to meet some new neighbours.

Harry and I went to church this morning and there was a special service about Max. The congregation wrote their thoughts about Max on post-it notes and the notes were all collected. Very moving, but managed to hold it together.

Harry and I then decided to travel the scenic route to Newcastle, up to Carlisle, stopping at Tebay Services on the way, and then across to Newcastle. A bit further but we were there in 3.5 hours.

It was lovely to be reunited with Max. He is on great form and we had a lovely time with him. Typing this in Scott House. Very tired, but ready for a week in Newcastle without work.

"So lovely to hear your posts, Emma. Thank you. So many positive results! Keep on doing what you're doing because it's *working well for you all. That heart has to come soon now – we're all praying for it! Love n light. Sue and Kath xx."*

"Wonderful news all round, Emma. It is so good that you have a couple of weeks to chill and spend precious time with your boys. I shall keep praying that a new heart for Max turns up very soon and that it will bring him the new life he so deserves. My love and prayers to you all xxx, Wendy."

"What a fantastic, heartrending message to us, Emma. We are so fortunate that you give the time to share with us everything you do with the family. It's great that Max seems now set up for hopefully that new heart waiting for him. So glad you enjoyed that precious time with Paul and Harry. What a wonderful family you all are. Love to super Max and to Harry and Paul and wonderful you. Malcolm and Sue xxx."

"Sounds as though a good week has been had by all from this week's really positive update! So pleased that Max's weight has improved and stabilised. Looks as though you packed a lot in whilst you were in Winsford this week, Emma! The garden party sounds as though it was a huge success and it was great that Max could be involved as well. That must have been fun. Our thoughts and prayers are with you as always. Love to you all, Jane and Bob x."

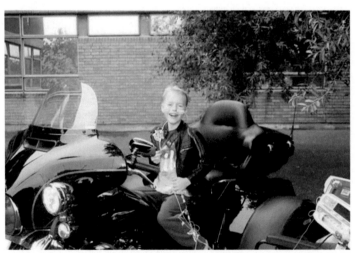

Max distracted from his feeding tube, with a visit by the Harley Davidson
Geordie Chapter.
Photo Credit: Emma Johnson

Chapter 10

Amongst people we knew, perhaps the hardest reaction to deal with was pity. Somehow, this made us feel as though our situation was hopeless, underpinned by the unspoken
"Thank God it's not us this is happening to!" Even harder was a wall of silence, "We haven't been in touch because we wouldn't know what to say." This made us feel lonely, because if other people didn't know what to say, then how did we begin to function? The reactions that were most comforting and gratefully received were; empathy, the offering of practical support and keeping us up-to-date with other people's news and activities, which proved a welcome distraction. We were so lucky that our friends and family almost exclusively played a blinder.

The longer the wait, the stronger a feeling of 'agonising yearning' for everything to be back to normal and for a future together in Cheshire as a healthy, fully-functioning family. For Emma, the feeling was almost physical and when hit by it, her jaw began to ache and she would feel light-headed. Only a good cry back at our room in Scott House could ease this pain; pent up emotion needs a release, like an overflowing dam. Emma tried to shield herself from this. She explained to me that it was as if she had an inner core that was one of misery and suffering for Max's plight and for the loss of our family life, but she had to pack the core with cotton wool to protect herself. Every so often, the inner core would leak and the cotton wool would get thin, soggy and saturated. That's when the overwhelming sadness hit her. We were suffering together, and yet our pain was also very personal.

She coped by convincing herself that for the time being, hospital life was our normality. Emma had recently started power walking one hour a day along the river in Freeman Park near the hospital. She would usually walk to Pets Corner and then walk back up the hill. It was only when she stopped and looked at the animals and other families with children enjoying their day out, that it hit her how much Max would love this and that what we were going through was so abnormal and unlucky.

When we were on the ward with Max, we tried to keep the mood cheerful and light to help him. We used humour and we sought to be positive. This wasn't always possible, as we were not infallible, but that was our goal. It was always lovely when Max would break out into laughter about some silly joke or prank. Early on during his time in Newcastle, the night shift reported for duty. By this stage, Max had already started to bond with some of the nurses, and one with whom he had such a bond walked into the High Dependency Unit to start her shift. With a smile on his face and a twinkle in his eye, Max said as bold as brass, "Oh no, not you again!"

It felt as if our role was to augment any silver lining around the indubitably black cloud, which hung menacingly over our world.

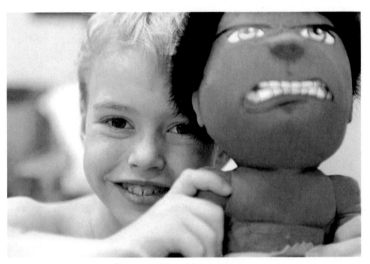

Max and his positive nature
Photo Credit: Marcus Taylor

Another powerful feeling was nostalgia; a longing to return to what we had been doing the same time the previous year. For example, the summer before, we had joined Winsford Tennis Club as a family and were loving playing tennis and watching Wimbledon together. A year later, Max and Emma watched the men's singles final in the ward playroom, charging up his various machinery batteries, whilst Harry and I were over in Cheshire. These kinds of memories emphasised how much our world had been turned upside down. When we were playing tennis in such a carefree way, we could never have anticipated what was about to happen to Max and our family.

Whilst we had been waiting for a new heart for Max, Emma found herself setting goals such as, 'Oh, if he gets his new gift by the end of May, then he can go back to school in September'. But then, when the self-imposed deadline passes, it felt soul-destroying, until you set a new goal such as, 'Oh, he will get his new gift over the summer and start school in January'. Emma knew she shouldn't really do this, as it was setting herself up for disappointment, but she just couldn't help it. Otherwise, the waiting would feel indefinite.

Max is an O blood group, which is unfavourable, because O hearts can be universal donors to any recipient blood type, so they tend to be spread thinly. However, an O recipient can only take the heart of an O blood group person. During our wait for Max's transplant, it was impossible to plan ahead, and so it felt like we were in an unnatural limbo land. Our dysfunctional life being marked off one day at a time; we could do nothing more and in any case, each day was a bonus and it may just be the day that a special little gift arrived.

I had just got out of bed and showered when the phone rang. For over nine months, my mobile phone was in perpetual use – I never switched it off, even when it was charging. It was Harry. "Hi Dad, how are you?" he asked.

"I'm fine, love, thank you – this is an early call – how are you all doing?"

There was a pause and Harry replied, "I'll pass the phone to Mum." Immediately, I thought something was afoot. Surely, nothing terrible had happened; I don't think Emma would have put Harry on the phone to have to break the worst news imaginable. As Harry handed the phone to Emma, I replayed the very brief conversation I'd just had. Was there something – anything – in Harry's intonation and general delivery to give me a clue? As I had done so many times with the doctors and consultants, I was searching for something – perhaps a subtext, a 'read the air' meaning – but I could find nothing.

"Hi, love," said Emma, "Max has an offer of a heart."

"Really?" I replied. I had been waiting for this moment for months – I knew it was his only chance of a life – but the swirling emotions had immediately begun and my mind was already trying to corral them so that I could begin to comprehend the impact of this news.

"I had the call in the middle of the night – if it goes ahead, it will be around half past one when he goes to theatre. Could you make your way up and be here by then?"

"Of course I can – how is Max?"

"He's fine, seems pretty relaxed."

"Okay, love, I'd better get myself ready and head off – I'll come up the M6, I think…okay. Love you and love to Harry and Max…bye." I pressed the red button on my handset and burst into tears.

My emotions had managed to corral themselves and I felt scared. One would think that excitement and relief would be at the forefront of my mind, but actually, I cried because I was scared. Max meant the world to us and we were now – if things went to plan and the operation took place – about to embark upon a one-way journey; there was no turning back. Max was about to receive his definitive treatment. If this didn't work, then that was it; game over and nothing to play for. I also, at this point, thought of a family somewhere, grieving the loss of a loved one, who had made or supported the bravest, most heroic decision one can make; to do something which saves the life of another.

In the months Max had been waiting, the consensus amongst the professionals treating him was that his wait had been unusually long; but by no means the longest. Now, on this Friday at the end of July, the wait was potentially over and our future would be decided over the ensuing hours. I packed, feeling a little numb, and took the car for fuel; it was 191 miles to Newcastle, and I didn't want to stop unless I – or Mother Nature – decided I needed to.

As I headed north up the M6 and into Cumbria, the monoliths which lined the route purveyed a sense of foreboding; dark, steep slopes, blotched with scree, they were a metaphor for the mountain we were about to climb. As the M6 finally discharged its duty, and with a ninety-degree turn became the A69, I had to stop. I found a burger van by the side of the road, adjacent to a railway line, and ordered a bacon and egg sandwich with a cup of tea, extra sugar. I sat behind the wheel of my car – I was making good progress – I was about an hour away from the hospital that was to represent the page onto which our family's destiny would be scribed. I sat and looked out of the window at the railway line disappearing to destination unknown; just like our lives. In my mind's eye, I played out various outcomes. I tried desperately hard to indelibly etch a positive, uplifting script line into the images I was conjuring, but there was nothing long lived about this craved for vista. As with the flame-like phosphorescence of will-o-the-wisp, the images failed to ignite into permanence. I couldn't finish my sandwich – I wasn't as hungry as I at first thought. I took a deep breath. Here we go. I rejoined the carriageway and headed into Newcastle, my stomach becoming increasingly knotted with the passage of each mile.

I pulled into the multi-storey car park early afternoon – the journey had taken some three hours and forty minutes. I hadn't rushed; my steady speed perhaps reflecting a reticence I was feeling. As I left the car and headed for the rotating door at the main entrance, my phone rang; it was Emma. "Hi Love, where are you?"

"I've literally just arrived and I'm walking into the building."

"Ah, okay…I'm afraid the operation is not going to take place. The heart was not functioning correctly on the journey. They'd used the 'heart in a box' and it started to go wrong, so they are not risking it. I'm afraid the heart was no good." I stopped in my tracks and just looked at the ground, letting Emma's words sink in. A huge swell of emotion swept over me; crushing sadness that Max was to remain in oblivion bound limbo, but also undeniable relief that I did not have to kiss him goodbye, never knowing if I'd see him again.

For the one thousandth time, I made my way along the Magnolia Mile to Max, Emma and Harry. On the ward, Max was putting a brave face on things, saying, "It wasn't meant to be – I didn't feel ready." Post-rationalising his disappointment, he was once again demonstrating that maturity, which belied his tender years. Nurses on the ward exchanged empathising words and looks with us; they had seen this numerous times before, but the gravity of this experience for our family was in no way lost on them. It was at this point that Neil Seller, one of the consultants, came over to us. He reassured us with his tone and certainty that the heart had not been suitable and that it was a complete non-starter. However, he could see through Max's valiant efforts at portraying a stiff upper lip; he knew that deep down he would be hurting and disappointed. The following day – and on a day off – Neil brought his two lovely sons onto the ward to play with Max and Harry. What a gentleman.

I believe in life that you should speak as you find, and what I found was a team of wonderful people, dedicated to the care of their patients, who thought nothing of putting themselves out, if it was felt that to do so would bring comfort, happiness and relief to the people in their care.

This weekend also saw a visit from Max's Granny, Grandpa and Uncle Marcus. Max has always been described as a bit of a Marcus in miniature, so he shares a close bond with his Uncle. It was Marcus who gave Max his old SLR camera, which proved to be such a wonderful distraction for Max and yielded some stunning photographs. When they left on the Monday morning, I couldn't help but notice that Uncle Marcus lingered with his hug and seemed reluctant to leave Max. Did he know something we didn't?

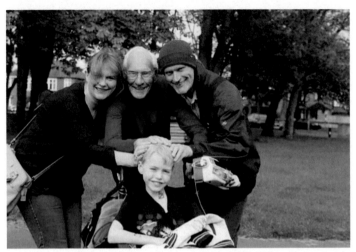

Max with Emma, Grandpa and Uncle Marcus
Photo Credit: Nurse Sophie

I left for Cheshire with Harry after lunch, promising to be back with Max at the weekend. We settled into the return journey, wondering about what might have been, but thanking our lucky stars that the potential donor heart had malfunctioned before it had been placed into Max's chest. We arrived home in Cheshire and after Harry had gathered a few clothes together, I dropped him for a sleepover with a friend. A bite of dinner and a 'personal' bottle (one glass only) of wine later, I was ascending the wooden hills to sleep...perchance to dream.

DIARY OF A HEART MUM: Twenty-Eighth Weekly Update – Sunday, 30 July 2017.

Quite a difficult week. The ward was extremely busy and quite noisy and there was little time for nurses to take Max out for wheelchair walks in the fresh air. So, we felt quite trapped and claustrophobic.

Harry tried a local sports camp on the Monday, but he just didn't enjoy it, so we let him miss the other days, but he got a viral infection and was confined to the adolescent room, so that he didn't come into contact with Max. I split my time dotting between Harry and Max. Quite stressful and frustrating!

Also, Scott House feeling crowded at the moment, so I avoided the communal areas, as really haven't felt like 'small talk' with other families. Really miss using the communal lounge occasionally and watching TV on a nice big screen, but it's never free these days. All this made me feel very confined. Max and I also managed to get stuck in the ward bathroom for 15 minutes as the lock broke and the utilities team practically had to break the door down to get us out! Was worried about Max's batteries draining or if he had a funny turn and the nurses would not be able to reach him.

The big news of the week was on Friday, when I got a call to say that the transplant coordinator had rung to confirm that a compatible heart had been found for Max and that he should be 'nil by mouth' and Paul should drive over from Cheshire. So, now we know how it feels to be told that the transplant might be going ahead. Harry and I quickly rushed down to the ward where Max was also told. We were told that, whilst looking promising, the operation could fall through at any stage. Max had bloods taken and we wheeled him off for a CT Scan, which he loved! ("Oooh, I could be transported through the portal to a parallel universe!") He said he was 'excited but nervous' about the transplant. The surgeon came to talk with me, and once again explained the risks etc. He also explained that the new heart would be transferred using 'heart in a box' technology. This enables the heart to keep beating on its journey to the recipient hospital.

Paul arrived in Newcastle, but by 15:00, we were told by the transplant coordinator, that she was really sorry, but that the transplant was not going to happen as the new heart wasn't working properly. Max took this really well, and surprisingly, so did we! We took some time to think about an unknown family who had lost their child, and who, at their worst moment of personal loss, had agreed to organ donation. How terribly sad and wonderful. Max spent about ten minutes staring at his 'Tree of Life', which is what he calls the tree outside his hospital window. He watches the leaves in the wind when he feels sad. I sat and held him. There were no words! Max was soon back to his perky self. Quite incredible!

On Saturday, Max finally got a walk in Freeman Park and we watched the miniature steamboats on the lake. Paul and I had CPR training back on the ward and we were finally given *permission to take Max off the ward without a nurse escort. This will make a huge difference to us all. Mum, Dad and Marcus arrived and we went to The Victory for dinner. It was lovely, but couldn't help wishing that the transplant the previous day had gone ahead.*

Max had managed to procure a small plastic doll's hand, and has taken great delight in pranking nurses by saying, "Do you need a hand?" and, "Don't worry, it's 'armless!"

Oh, well...after such a difficult week, I have to somehow muster the energy to return to work tomorrow! Time for a glass of red wine and pizza tonight though!

"Wow, Em, what a difficult week for everyone. Goodness knows how you are getting through this turbulent time. Such a sad time for another family as you say, and a huge disappointment for you all this week, but hoping and praying that a new heart will soon be there for Max. Much love from us all, as always xx, Janis."

"What a week for you all, Emma. I am glad that Max coped well with the disappointment and retains his great sense of humour! I hope you managed to find the energy for today and things improve for you this week. Elaine xx."

"What a roller coaster of a week you have all had. You all show such bravery in the way you have dealt with the disappointment of the possible heart transplant not being viable. I feel sure the right one will turn up. So tough for all concerned. I suppose the hospital is busier because of the summer holidays. I know how you feel not wanting to 'chat' to other mothers. A normal life would be good. Never give up hope, dear Emma. I can tell you are a fighter, as you all are. Blessings and love, Wendy xxx."

"Wow, Emma, what an emotional week for you all. Friday must have been so difficult for you all to get so close to the transplant. Fingers crossed for next time. What a brave family who made the hard decision to donate their family member's organs. Hopefully, a more positive week for you all this week. Enjoy your wine and pizza. Sending lots of love to you all. Love. Vicky xxxx."

I had just finished dreaming about winning the Mr Olympia title (I have more chance of becoming our next king), when my mobile phone started to ring. The Samsung ringtone, which causes such confusion in public places as multiple people scramble for their phones upon hearing it, woke me almost immediately. I knew straight away that it was Emma and there must be some breaking news 191 miles away. I answered, "Hi, love, is everything okay?"

"Hi, love, you'll never guess…Max has had another offer of a heart…I've just spoken with Lisa on the ward. They've not woken him, as there is no point. If it happens, it will be half past two in the afternoon when he goes to theatre. Can you make your way up in the morning?"

"Of course, love – I'll pick Harry up and come straight away – first thing." I put the phone down, and feeling much calmer than I had on the previous occasion, I sought sleep once more. I set my alarm, but realised that I really wouldn't need it – sleep was going to be light and ephemeral.

I was up and ready to go by seven o'clock. I had a touch of breakfast and headed over to collect Harry from his friend's house. I had been unable to make contact, so I had to knock-on. A bleary-eyed Harry came to the door, but he woke up the second his sluggish synapses realised it was me standing there. "Is Max okay?" were the first words out of his mouth.

"He's fine, love, don't worry…unbelievably, he has another offer of a heart. Get your stuff together – I've got you some breakfast – we're off to Newcastle again." Harry distracted himself on the long journey with his 'screen' – this was the escapism, which helped him to cope with such tumult in his young life. We stopped at Tebay services for a sausage sandwich. I looked at all of the families going about their business. We were in peak holiday season, so the place was full of super dads in Rohan walking trousers and matching hiking boots, kids trailing behind them. I thought, *bloody hell, I'm travelling to my nine-year-old son, who is about to have a heart transplant.* It was such a contrast; the steady metre which identifies the background music of normal life, set against the arrhythmic beat of our life's current soundtrack.

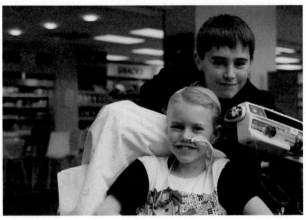

Max and Harry in the hospital cafe, two days before Max's heart
transplant
Photo Credit: Marcus Taylor

We arrived at the Freeman and again, we had made good time.
I felt a different vibe on this occasion – somehow the air was
charged and there was always a sense of 'things' happening behind
the scenes. During their wait for the previous offer to be confirmed,
Emma and Max had managed to get locked in the ward shower room.
It was at this point, Max claims, that he realised the transplant was
not going to happen. Even Emma felt that the episode – positively
comical, as the hospital handymen (Tommy Cooper and Bernard
Cribbins) tried to release them from their ablutionary prison – was
a bad omen. On this second occasion, there were no such episodes;
people visited Max's bed space with purpose and it was clear that
this time, it was looking good.

It was at around two o'clock when the transplant co-ordinator,
Alison, came to confirm that the transplant was going ahead and that
Max would be taken to theatre at around three. By this time, James
and Leanne had joined us. They were filming a BBC 2 documentary,
celebrating the fifty years that had elapsed since the first heart
transplant in South Africa. A lovely, respectful team, they had
filmed Max on numerous occasions, as he waited for his transplant.
We had agreed for them to film Max's transplant – when it came –
but it had looked like Max was not going to get his little gift before
the filming ended, and James and Leanne headed back to London
for good. They had travelled up the previous week and had been
ready to film the 'first' transplant. Now, they had made the journey

for a second time in almost as many days, in the hope that they would get the footage they so desperately wanted for Max's part of the story.

As we sat as a family of four and chatted, we played a game of Uno – again, Max applying his usual and somewhat unique interpretation of the rules. James was setting up the cameras in theatre, so Leanne discretely filmed us as we waited nervously for things to develop. Max stood on his bed and asked me for a hug. I stood and held him tight, his soft blonde hair gently tickling my cheek. Max later confessed that he wanted the hug, as he feared it may be our last. What a thing for my beautiful nine-year-old son to be thinking. Heart breaking. About twenty minutes before he was taken to theatre, Max was given some medication, to help to detach him from the reality, nerves and outright worry of the situation. We knew from previous administering of this drug that it caused Max to become a little manic. We had been assured that he would not remember this – and he doesn't – but it was distressing to watch. Crying, laughing, shouting out or lying quietly; a veritable gamut of contrasting behaviours were teased out by this amnesia-inducing cocktail.

By now, we were preparing to head for theatre. There is some footage, taken by Leanne, which shows Max lying quietly on his bed as we began the move. It tugs at the heartstrings like little else. In those few seconds of footage, you see a small boy who looks scared, lost and so gut wrenchingly vulnerable – the proverbial rabbit in the headlights of a car. Again. When he was taken to surgery for his LVAD to be fitted, Max didn't truly appreciate what was about to happen to him; how could he? Now, though, he had a frame of reference and the enormity of what he was about to go through was not lost on him. Vikki, one of the play specialists, had joined us and was doing a brilliant job of calming and supporting Max. As we left the ward to head for theatre, I put my arm around Harry's shoulders. He would not be allowed into the theatre complex, so he would be saying goodbye to Max very soon. I so desperately wanted to reassure him – for Harry to know that we were there for him – not just Max.

As we entered the doors to theatre, we said goodbye to Harry who went to the ward with one of the nurses and we put our ill-fitting (in my case, at least) theatre gowns on. Leanne was continuing to film, as one of the team came to confirm that Max was, indeed, Max and to finalise administrative matters. By this stage, Max was singing at full tilt, 'My Heart Skips a Beat' by Olly Murs.

I don't think that the irony was lost on any of us. Both Emma and I fought back our tears – it was so hard – but we didn't want to give Max any cause for additional worry. I nearly bit through my lip, but as I was standing just behind Max's line of sight, I knew he couldn't see me. Emma stroked Max's head. After a few minutes, the doors opened and we made our way along the sterile corridor and into the same theatre Max had been in for his LVAD operation. I noticed four very discrete cameras positioned around the operating table and saw again the machine that would keep Max alive – this time when his chest didn't have a heart in it. Max continued in his manic ways, but was now whimpering – his big blue eyes wide open as his addled consciousness tried to comprehend what was happening. Soothing platitudes from the theatre team and anaesthetist did more to calm us, I think, and maybe that was the intention! I felt light-headed – I knew that my emotions were building with intense pressure – they would need a release, but not just yet. As before, the anaesthetic was administered slowly. Incredibly, just before he fell asleep, Max became completely lucid, and perhaps in a moment of scared realisation, said: "It will be a while until I see you again. I love you both."

"We love you too, Max," and as we said this, his beautiful eyes closed and he was gone. I kissed his forehead, whispered to him that I loved him and turned to leave the theatre.

As I walked through the double doors and away from Max, I let out a doleful cry and tears cascaded down my cheeks. My emotion could be contained no more. I knew that there was a twenty percent chance that I would never see Max again – I had lived with these Damoclean odds for months – but the reality of that situation and what it meant floored me. I felt sick and overwhelmed with grief. *Please, God, bring him home.*

At the entrance to the theatre complex, I sat and slowly regained my composure. Emma, too, had found the experience as challenging as I. To the left of me were bags of O-negative blood, with Max's name on them. Not only had some hero donated the organ of a loved one; other heroes had taken time to give lifesaving blood. Without them, this operation would not be taking place. We made our way back down to the ward and picked up Harry. As ever, the staff team were so kind, arms around shoulders and kind words, "Get out of here and try to relax. We'll call you if we need you." Alison, our transplant co-ordinator, said that things would probably all be finished at around 00:15. The wait had begun.

We headed to the health club across the road from the hospital. So often one of our boltholes, we sat and had some dinner, soaking up the surreal feelings we were experiencing. What little appetite we had satiated, we slowly ambled back to Scott House, every so often, checking our watches and trying to second-guess what was happening to Max. Naturally, we had no idea. We surfed and watched television, paying scant regard to the screens before our eyes, and then amazingly, we decided to try and drop off to sleep. Incredibly, we managed it.

Chapter 11

It was 00:15 when the phone rang – exactly the time the transplant co-ordinator had said it would.

The piercing, 'wake the dead' tone jolted us from our restless sleep. "Hi," said the voice, "it's PICU here – Max is back from theatre and they're just setting him up – do you want to make your way over?" My mind raced with questions, "How did it go?" and, "Is he okay?" but such questions could wait…our son had a new heart beating in his chest and he'd made it through the surgery.

We quickly dressed and made our way out into the fast cooling summer night. In the darkness, the bright lights of the hospital drew us towards our son and his new heart. We started our walk along the Magnolia Mile – the long corridor running through the hospital like an artery. Tonight, it was deserted, our footsteps our only company, our hearts pounding in our ears.

For months at the end of the corridor, we had turned right into Ward 23 and the High Dependency Unit, which had been our second home. Tonight, we turned left and climbed the stairs which would take us to the Paediatric Intensive Care Unit and our little boy. Pushing the 'buzzer', we looked at one another and took a deep breath. "Hello, can I help?"

"It's Max's Mum and Dad."

"Just a minute." We paused, wondering if we would be instructed to wait in the family room, hoping, praying that we would not.

"Okay, come in." came the response, and the door gave its customary squeak as the magnetic lock relented to grant us entry.

We washed our hands and put on our plastic aprons. Infection is the biggest risk when people visit transplanted patients, so it was vital that we did everything we could to minimise that risk. We walked down the corridor and onto the ward. In the semi-darkness, machines whizzed and beeped, tubes and wires, branching like trees, all had their common meeting point; a small child or baby, whose heart needed help.

Sitting behind the desk as we rounded the corner, was the gentle, softly spoken and quite brilliant surgeon, Fabrizio de Rita who, along with Mr Asif Hasan and his team, had successfully fitted our son's 'little gift'. Our surgeon sat, coolly looking at his phone – he seemed relaxed, but his eyes looked tired. We were shown into a side room, along the corridor which lead to the cubicles and our son.

We sat down and waited for the surgeon and nurses to come and brief us. I had been in this room before, during the darker days of Max's time at the Freeman. I had cried, as I talked to the psychologist about my fears for Max's prospects of getting a new heart – of being well enough and strong enough to get a new heart. I had also thought of the parents who had sat in the same, red vinyl seat as me, being given the news that every parent dreads. Tonight, and at this moment, it seemed that the update might…dare I say or even think it…be good.

As I finished scanning the leaflets on the opposite wall – each one carrying its own devastating assessment of what can go wrong with the heart – the door opened. In walked the surgeon. In his lilting Italian tone, Fabrizio informed us that the operation had gone well, that the heart was good and that everything had gone to plan. I waited for the 'but'…surely, there must be a 'but'! Not on this occasion. The next 24 hours would be critical, but as we sat in that room at around twenty to one in the morning, it seemed we had much to be cautiously optimistic about.

Upon being shown into Max's cubicle, the enormity of the situation hit home. We had been told that his chest may be open, or that he may be on the ECMO machine. Neither possibility was welcome, especially the latter, as this would mean that the new heart was not working properly and needed help; if this were the case, then the sands of time were made up of an alarmingly small number of grains. Thankfully, Max's chest was closed, and save for three large drains coming out of his abdomen, he was suitably contained.

Max had a breathing tube coming out of the right corner of his mouth. His chest and abdomen were covered with wires – some with which we were entirely familiar, yet others, like his 'pacing wires' (or 'jump leads' as we called them) were clearly new and specific to the operation he had had. Many relatives of heart transplant patients talk of how red the recipient looks after surgery; their lips full and flushed. However, Max just looked really pale, so fragile and beaten – for one so young, having been through such an ordeal. I looked at the banks of IV machines, filling his blood stream with numerous medications to prevent infection and rejection, whilst helping the new heart get used to its new home. I glanced at the monitor – his heart was beating a solid, unwavering 120 beats per minute (bpm); a stark contrast to his old heart, which could range from 140 bpm whilst at complete rest, to 150 plus bpm if he so much as moved his position. What a difference!

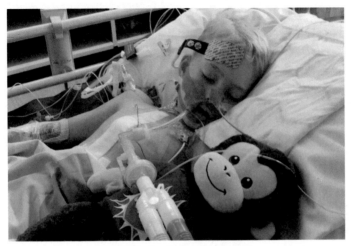

Max just after his heart transplant
Photo Credit: Emma Johnson

We stayed only a few minutes, wanting to let the team of nurses carry on with their unstinting care of our son. As we left, I looked at the notice board on the wall in the cubicle. On it was written Max's name in shadow writing and underneath it, was a heart with a little arrow through it. Beneath was the signature of the artist – the surgeon, Fabrizio, who had transplanted our son. In that moment, the sheer majesty and beauty of the care Max was under, became so clear in my mind – in the months that he had been in hospital, the nameless acts of kindness and love bestowed by all of the staff had made the essence of his care somehow greater than the sum of its parts.

Underpinning all of this was a thought that struck me as I watched Max's chest, rising and falling in time with his ventilator and it has stayed with me ever since. Somewhere, possibly in Europe, but almost certainly in the UK, was a family grieving for the loss of a priceless child, who had made all of this possible; whose humanity and courage at the darkest, coldest and saddest time in their lives had given our son a chance of life. Their child's

'Golden Heart' was now beating in Max's chest, a part of him and a part of us…it is thanks to them that we were standing next to our son who now had a future, but there were times when we honestly thought we would never make it. That Willow Tree 'Heart of Gold' figurine had a new symbolic significance.

We returned to Scott House, having only spent ten minutes with Max. He was still out for the count and we just didn't want to hamper the intensive care he required. Sleep for us was out of the question, so we turned to that time-honoured British remedy for stressful situations; a nice sweet cup of tea. Okay, not an ideal thing to be imbibing at two o'clock in the morning, but the events of the previous twenty-four hours were of too great a magnitude to just be able to switch off. It was an incredible feeling to be able to tell Harry that his brother had made it over yet another hurdle – yes, the next couple of days would be critical – but at least the little man had battled through the biggest challenge to date of his young life.

We sat in silence in our room, slowly sipping our soothing elixir. Tonight, another chapter had been opened in our family life, and although the ink was still wet, the first paragraph had been committed to the page successfully. Let us hope, I thought to myself, that the book containing this and subsequent chapters would be long and involve all four of us. The following morning, we were up at eight o'clock. We had agreed that we would take it in turns to be with Max and Harry respectively. At this early stage, only the parents are allowed into the cubicle, to minimise the risk of any infection. Immediately after his transplant, Max's immune system was pretty well wiped out, so that his body did not rally to reject his new heart; a foreign body, as far as his immune system was concerned. Therefore, one entered the cubicle through an anteroom, which contained unused items of cubicle paraphernalia and a sink, for those entering and leaving to wash their hands. Hand washing and general cleanliness was vital at this stage, and to this day, it remains extremely important. A dose of norovirus for Max would have been a disaster.

Documentary makers James and Leanne popped up to the ward to video Max 'the morning after the night before' and Emma happened to be in the cubicle. In the finished documentary, Heart Transplant: A Chance to Live (BBC 2, 19/05/2018, 2100hrs), a short interview with Emma is shown which was recorded during this brief visit. In it, Emma makes reference to Max starting to exercise his personality again, with arm gestures and flourishes, which seemed to succinctly communicate approval and irritation; so Max. What I can see – and doubtless those that know Emma – is how tired she looks. There is no escaping the stress and tension this situation had wrought; it was inescapably manifest in the lines on our faces and bags under our eyes. It was also indelibly marked on our souls – the experience had changed us.

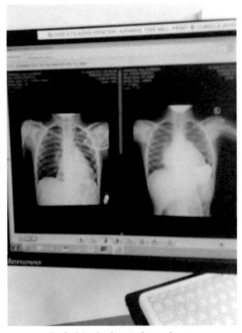

Left: Max's donated new heart.
Right: Max's old, enlarged heart with mechanical pump.
Photo Credit: Emma Johnson

Already, Max was starting to come back online; the reboot was in full swing. By the end of day one, the ventilator tube was out, and he was breathing on his own. For months, Max had been unable to breathe properly. His failing heart had damaged everything; generally, his breathing was much faster than normal and very shallow. As a consequence, the bottom quarter or so of his right lung had simply collapsed. The team treating Max was very keen to resolve this issue, as 'dead' space at the bottom of his lung could be a breeding ground for bacteria and infection. To help, he was placed back on the 'Vapotherm' machine, which pumped air under pressure up into Max's nostrils, mixed with water, to stop his nose from becoming sore. Max simply hated this machine. When he'd needed

165

it around early March to help his then broken heart, he had placed tissues under his nose to catch the water spray from the machine. The tissue hung down in front of his mouth, making him look like a Bedouin tribeswoman! Max did not see the funny side, and I can understand this; it was not his choice.

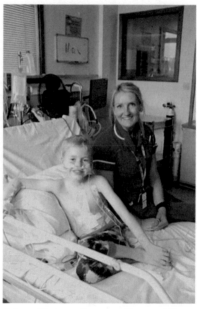

Max with transplant coordinator, Alison
Photo Credit: Emma Johnson

One of the first things Max said to Emma when he woke up was "I can see clearly". I guess we think of heart failure as being something which stops you walking very far, or makes you short of breath. And it does. However, it impacts much more than that. As we have chatted about our experience with Max in the months since he returned home, it is clear that his senses were being dimmed by an inadequate blood supply from his broken heart. Numbness in his hands and fingers, poor eyesight and a diminishing sense of smell – it's like the functions of a computer slowly failing as the battery runs out. Now, Max reported twenty/twenty vision, perfect smell and touch – how true that you don't know what you've got until it's gone.

After a few days, Harry was allowed into the cubicle anteroom, but not fully into the cubicle. This worked initially, as the two brothers were able to share smiles, air kisses and just enjoy the fact that they were both together in this world. After a while, though, it became frustrating for Harry to be stuck in this necessary limbo land, so his visits were managed to be concise yet reassuring for both boys. Max had a regime of breathing exercises to undertake in order to get that slacking quadrant of lung working again. It was feared that due to his 'lazy lung', he had contracted pneumonia, but luckily, this fear proved unfounded. Once more, I started to get notifications on my phone – usually in the morning – that Max was launching a counterattack on one of his favourite games, so I knew that he was feeling increasingly more of sorts.

Emma and I had, the morning after the transplant, notified close family and friends that Max had been transplanted. I had called my father as Max was in theatre, asking him to pray for his grandson. At the time of my call, he was looking after Max's cousins and they were listening to a recording of my Dad's favourite hymn (Love Divine All Loves Excelling, to the tune Blaenwern), which we had played at Mum's funeral. What timing. My Dad wept as I told him the news.

DIARY OF A HEART MUM: Twenty-Ninth Weekly Update – Sunday, 6 August 2017.

THIS WAS THE WEEK THAT WAS!

Max has a new heart! The 2nd August will be forever etched into our family calendar! The call came at 2:30 am. "The transplant coordinator just called to say that we have a potential heart for Max!" Paul and Harry left Cheshire at 8 am and arrived just after 12:00.

Max was prepped through the morning, but we didn't know for sure that the transplant would definitely happen until 14:30. At 15:00, Max was given 'premed' medication to make him relaxed. Boy, it certainly had an effect on him; he lurched from shouting out, to tearful, to giggly, to singing, to lucid and back to shouting again. Really difficult to witness! Although his rendition of Olly Murs' 'My heart skip skips a beat' caused much amusement!

We went in to the operating theatre with him. His last words to us before dropping to sleep were, "I might not see you for a while! I love you both!" We were in bits when we walked out!

The next dilemma is how do you pass the time whilst your son is having open-heart surgery! We decided to wander over to David Lloyd for a cup of tea, sitting on comfy sofas in a nice private corner. We were still in there by 18:00, so we had some tea and we succumbed to a glass of red wine! We wandered back to Scott House, and by 22:00, we felt so tired and drained that we all managed to drop off. The phone rang at quarter past midnight! Max was out and we could come over. The heart surgeon met us and explained that everything had gone smoothly and that there were no complications. We were told that Max's old heart was huge and that the new heart was excellent. Double-edged sword, as a family has lost a child. We are so indebted to the family for agreeing to organ donation.

We went in to see Max; oh, the tubes and wires! This time, the nappy Max had to wear reminded me of rebirth – a new beginning – a second chance, rather than regression.

Max got through the first critical 48 hours very successfully. His breathing tube was removed on Thursday, and the catheter and neckline removed on Friday. He is very fragile and overwhelmed, but physically, he is doing really well, with just a bit of congestion in the right lung, which the chest physios are dealing with. The care is just brilliant!

"Emma, we've just come back from holiday to this amazing news. Wonderful! Congratulations! I hope everything is going well and praying for Max and you all that everyone continues to stay well and that Max improves day by day. Fantastic news. With all our love and best wishes. Maria."

"Amazing news! We are all so pleased, lots of love and hugs to you all from all the staff at Nationwide Winsford xxx."

"Great news, Emma – here's to a wonderful summer for you all now! Lots of love, Margaret."

"Just…wonderful. I had a message from Irene Walker (nee Barnard) and also her Mum in South Africa. Both delighted at the news and wishing Max as speedy a recovery as possible. Both added that they are very proud Barnards! Liz C."

"Oh, what brilliant news. I've been busy phoning folks you will never know but who have added Max's name to the prayer lists in different churches. You have been so very brave during the last months. So pleased that the recovery is going well and hope he will soon be well again and able to enjoy so many things he has been missing. Love to you all, Gill and Lewis."

"Oh, Emma, the greatest of news. Like many of the other posts – I'm in tears reading this. So glad to hear that it all seemed to go *well, and wishing Max a speedy and complete recovery. Lots of love to you all, Nick, Penny, Zoe and Emily."*

"Amazing news, also crying here! Are you able to personally thank your donor family or is the donation anonymous? So fantastic that his recovery is going so well. Bless Harry, it's difficult to express thoughts and feelings at his age and the emotions that go with a six-month long process like this are complex and huge! But he has coped so well and you must be so proud of them both. I LOVE that Max was singing 'My heart skips a beat'! Love to you all, and hope to see you soon xxxx, Ailsa."

"We are leaping up and down with joy! Fantastic news, Emma. Love to all! Xxx Tears and tears! Malcolm."

"Thrilled to hear your fantastic news this week, and that Max is doing so well. Love to you all, Jane and Bob xxx."

"Crying! Ben."

"In tears also! But ecstatic for you all! Thanks so much, Em, for taking the time to share all this with us. Sending much love as always from all the Finnigans xx."

"I am in tears reading this. Thank you for sharing. Lots of love as always to you all. Xxxx Vicky."

"Absolutely thrilled to hear this news! Lots of love to you all xxxxx, Elaine."

"What fantastic news, and brought tears to my eyes. Glad you can all be together to get through this part. Take care. Thinking of you all. Say hi to Harry for us and we must take him biking again sometime soon. Nic and Tracey."

As each day came anew, Max made progress. On a couple of occasions, there were bumps in the road (blood and pacing wire infections), but the direction of travel was undeniably positive – we knew we were very lucky. After eight days, Max was deemed well enough to make the trip downstairs to a side room on Ward 23.

As he was wheeled through the intensive care unit, the nurses looked delighted…not to be getting rid of him, of course…but to see him looking so much stronger and hopefully on the road to recovery. How it must break their hearts when it doesn't pan out like that. When Max was rolled into Ward 23, he started to cry. Emma asked him if he was okay, with Max replying, "I'm so happy!" He was back in familiar, safe and reassuring territory. Max was still on Milrinone at this point, albeit a much-reduced dose to the one he had been on before his operation. His new heart was – as apparently many transplanted hearts are – impaired on the right side; something to do with the timing of events as the little gift is recovered. I had developed a real love/hate relationship with this drug. On the one hand, it had supported Max's failing heart when it most needed it, bringing him back from the brink. On the other hand, his utter dependence on this drug confirmed the gravity of his situation, and thus, the only course of action that could put things right. So, for me, the day he was free from Milrinone would be a good day.

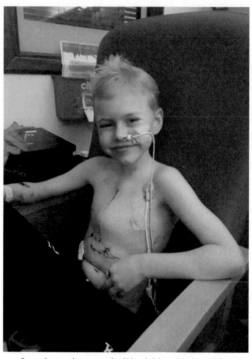

Max down from intensive care in Ward 23 cubicle, with colour in his cheeks
Photo Credit: Emma Johnson

Ensconced in his side room, in a location where the nurses could keep their eyes on him (always a good move), Max set about personalising his space. First of all, he set up his sound systems – yes, he had more than one. Then the disco light was positioned to yield the most effusive lightshow possible – surprisingly, a critical element in helping Max capture sleep. Finally, his bed was made using his own duvet set. For the first time in months, he had something approximating a private space, which he was well enough to be able to enjoy. At last, Harry was allowed to enter the room and the two boys could hug; a simple act, but one which can convey so much; love, protection, warmth, gratitude and safety.

As the days passed, Max was able to venture out into the corridor when the coast was clear. To be able to walk up and down, feeling strong and in control was an incredible feeling. Imagine, then, his joy when the Milrinone was finally switched off. For the first time in nine months, he was an independent human being, free from any shackles – he could run up and down the corridor – heck, he could turn 360 degrees.

Every morning at 0800hrs, we had to be on the ward to administer his medication. No longer could we rely upon the nurses to medicate Max – we needed to get used to what this was like ahead of our discharge and return home. Needless to say, there were quite a few. Cyclosporin, Prednisolone, Azathioprine, Furosemide, Aciclovir – the list was long. We would use Max's tray to prepare the concoctions, after which two nurses would come and check for mistakes; at this point, we still needed 'top cover' to prevent and detect errors, as we got used to this new and critical requirement of us. In one of the transplant information leaflets, it did make the point that a failure to take medication would 'invariably result in death'. No pressure there, then. At two o'clock in the afternoon, further medication was administered, followed by the last dose at 2000hrs. Max will be required to take anti-rejection medication twice a day for the rest of his life. This is non-negotiable, for the reasons concisely outlined above.

Finally, it felt like we could relax a little bit. We enjoyed several meals at The Victory and we both took Harry on day trips; this was his summer holiday, after all. After a couple of weeks in the side room, which had been accompanied by continuing bouts of physiotherapy for his breathing and to address muscle atrophy, Max was given the green light to move to the 'transplant flat' in Scott House. This stupendous facility just kept on giving. The transplant flat is a self-contained dwelling within Scott House that allows families to be together – in our case, for the first time in nine months – to get used to life as a family with a transplanted child. Psychologically, this was very important; to know you were within touching distance of the ward was very reassuring and one cannot underestimate how much adjusting needed to be done. Furthermore, there were a couple of occasions where being close to the ward was actually vital.

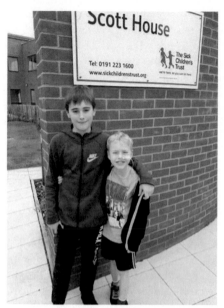

Max and Harry, outside Scott House
Photo Credit: Paul Johnson

One Sunday morning, just before his move to Scott House, Max and I had been sitting in his room together. Max, unsurprisingly, was launching another of those counter attacks and I was drifting in and out of consciousness on the 'big' chair. All of a sudden, his vital signs monitor started binging, ramping things up to a shriek within a couple of seconds. It did this as the gravity of the unfolding vital signs issue became more pronounced. I turned and looked at the screen. Max's pulse was at 180 beats per minute. As I watched the monitor, the number started to fall, back to around 115 beats per minute. Max told me that he had felt his heart racing, so this was not a faulty reading. A nurse came into the room and I relayed what had happened; she left to find one of the doctors. Again, the machine started shrieking as Max's pulse raced to 185 beats per minute. I was getting worried, and although Max remained outwardly cool, I could tell that this was disconcerting for him. His pulse then settled, but a few minutes later, it did the same thing and then again and again.

By this time, the 'A team' had arrived. Dr Reinhardt – our transplant consultant – and Andreas had taken up position in Max's cubicle and were cogitating about the possible cause. I can't remember if I made a contribution to the conversation, but if I did, I doubt my input was of any real value. I was just getting a little bit freaked out. These surges were happening with alarming regularity and not knowing the cause was very worrying. Andreas and Dr Reinhardt were able to take a reading from the vital signs monitor, even though a full ECG (Electrocardiogram) was commissioned as a matter of urgency. Looking at the data provided by Max's monitor, they identified some anomaly, which told them that Max was magnesium deficient; another one of those vital elements. Not for the first time during his stay in hospital, a large syringe of liquid – this time magnesium – was pumped into Max's body. One of the sisters, Kirsten, looked at me and said with a smile, "You're more worried than he (Max) is." – Yes, I think I was. Thanks to the magnesium and the quick thinking of Dr Reinhardt and Andreas, Max's little ticker settled down, but the incident confirmed the need to be in close proximity to help during these early stages of Max's recovery.

As time pressed onwards, an indication of Max's further progress was the gradual riddance of outward indications betraying his condition; his drugs, lines and wires. The departure of Milrinone from the scene meant that he was no longer accompanied by a drip stand and pump. When his heart was first transplanted, he had these fine blue wires emanating from the top of his abdomen. Called pacing wires – now renamed jump leads – they were initially attached to an external pace maker, in case the heart needed help with pace and rhythm. Amazingly, these wires, which were latterly tied off in a neat bow, were attached directly to Max's new heart and their removal – with some gas and air for Max – involved gently pulling them from their mooring on the wall of his heart. All that remained was his Alan Rickman; Hickman (line). To facilitate the removal of these tubes, he would need to be taken to theatre and given a general anaesthetic.

Max had already experienced a biopsy under general anaesthetic, which had seen a tiny sliver of heart muscle being taken to identify any signs of rejection; thankfully there were none, and they decided that the second biopsy, planned for a couple of weeks hence, was not required. Max's Alan Rickman was removed without issue and he spent the afternoon recovering with his Mum in Scott House. All was going well, until Max asked his Mum: "Is my heart supposed to do this?" Emma fixed Max with an intent gaze and asked him,

"What do you mean?"

Max said, "Have a feel." Emma managed to locate Max's pulse and it was undeniably irregular. What to do? Immediately, she called the ward and they instructed that Max be brought to them straight away. Sitting in his wheelchair, with his heart improvising a new kind of beat, a worried Emma conveyed Max to the ward. En route, they bumped into the enigmatic Mr Hasan. Emma explained what had happened, to which Mr Hasan gently took Max's wrist in his hand and quietly tuned in to the little man's heartbeat. With the calmness of deep, still waters, he said: "He has an irregular beat – take him to the ward straight away." During our time at the Freeman, we bore witness to a number of urgent medical interventions, but the staff always managed to portray the model of unflappable composure and quick thinking. Goodness only knows if their legs were like the proverbial swan, flailing away under the water; if they were, it never showed.

Arriving at the ward, Max was hooked up to a monitor and it immediately reproduced the little hiccup in his heartbeat. Not at all surprisingly, Mr Hasan's diagnosis was confirmed sometime later, verbatim. Max was kept in overnight, and as the night reached its zenith, his new little heart regained its sinusoidal rhythm once more. Again, thank goodness we were near to help when it was needed.

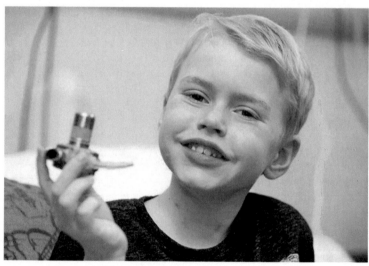

Max with his mechanical pump
Photo Credit: Andy Commins/Mirror Newspaper Group

During Max's convalescence in Scott House, Emma was allowed to take him on day trips away from the hospital. These were incredibly special times for Emma and Max. They could sit in a café, or walk around Hadrian's Wall and people they passed would have no idea what the little blonde boy, so full of life, had been through. Already, the magic of transplantation was making itself known. For Max, this was a taste of the freedom he had so longed for as he stared at the 'Tree of Life' from his bed in Ward 23. For Emma, she had been given back her son and at times, she would have to pinch herself; is this really happening? Emma will never forget the response of the Vicar and church friends from St Chad's Church to Max's illness and transplant. In one service, the congregation all wrote prayers for Max. The most common words were then collected and made into a picture for him. The bigger the word appeared on the page...the more it had appeared in the prayers. It was such a beautiful idea and is something that Max will treasure forever.

On the 14 September 2017, the go-ahead was given for Max to go home. He had been attending his weekly transplant clinic whilst still at the hospital, and the team felt that they had his condition at a place, conducive to his being discharged. Harry and I had been in Newcastle a few days prior to Max's departure and had packed the car with the accrued detritus of some nine months in hospital. This meant that the process of leaving the incredible transplant flat in Scott House would be so much easier. In any case, there would be another patient who would need it soon.

One abiding memory of this time is our first trip out as a complete family, with Max in tow, down to St Mary's Lighthouse. Our Newcastle rock (not to be mistaken for Blackpool rock), Norma, had prepared a gorgeous picnic for us. We were a little anxious, but it was lovely and incredibly moving to watch Max paddling in the sea and buried in sand after nine months stuck in hospital! Norma had made us feel at ease and we started to relax a little.

Max and Emma spent their last night in Newcastle with Norma and she helped them to meditate and welcome Max's new heart into his little body. "Send that lovely new heart all the love in the world!" To this day, Max does just that.

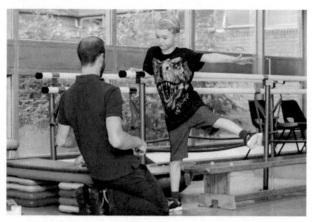
Max with his physiotherapist, just before being discharged.
Photo Credit: Andy Commins/Mirror Newspaper Group

Max and Emma said their goodbyes to the staff on the ward and the wonderful people at Scott House who'd looked after us so well. How can you begin to thank the team who had so skilfully saved your son's life and given him a second chance at achieving sixty seconds worth of distance run? Without exception, they had proven that their chosen career was, at its very heart, a true vocation. They had gone out of their way to make Max's time in hospital as comfortable and pain free as possible; both physically and psychologically. Not only that, they had managed to tread that fine line of kindness and engagement with professionalism when dealing with us, with such skill and judgement. Sometimes, you needed that little bit more from them, and they never failed to deliver; be it Neil Seller and his sons, or an embracing arm around a shoulder. Wonderful people doing an incredible job. So it was that Max and Emma set off for home – a wildest dream that at times seemed so far off as to be unattainable – was now a reality. *Thank you, thank you, thank you.*

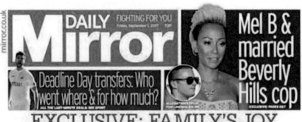

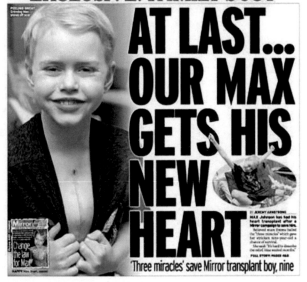

The Mirror reveals that Max has a new heart
Photo Credit: Andy Commins/Mirror Newspaper Group

Chapter 12

Max was discharged from the Freeman Hospital on 14 September 2017; over nine months since he was first admitted to Leighton Hospital on 8 December 2016. For a few days prior to discharge, Harry and I had been at home. Harry had started the new school term and we were determined to try to minimise further impact on his education.

Whilst at home, waiting for launch control to give the go ahead, I had busied myself finishing off the myriad DIY projects I had undertaken in preparation for the big day. Fitting these home improvement endeavours around my work commitments was not easy; not least because I am not a skilled DIYer. With the help of Max's Uncle Roger, I assembled Max's new bunk bed, which weighed a tonne and the instructions may as well have been written in Klingon. Taking photographs of an increasingly sweaty and frustrated me as the build progressed (slowly), I sent the images to Max for his perusal. What is so lovely with Max is that the arrival of these progress shots prompted a very sweet and heartfelt outpouring of gratitude on his part; there was no doubt in my mind that he really appreciated what was being done for him. *Good job,* I thought!

With the house cleaned for about the fifth time, word arrived that Max and Emma had set off from Newcastle. They would be avoiding motorway services to reduce the risk of catching an infection in what were still early days post-transplant. I had whipped into Winsford town to buy a 'Welcome Home' banner. Max and I had discussed, in some detail, the route he would take upon arrival; it will not surprise you to learn that his bedroom was to be the last room he would enter, and believe me, it had changed beyond recognition. Harry returned home from school and we nervously waited for the arrival of this most special little boy.

Emma and Max had taken a pit stop at Emma's parents' home and Max had run up and down the stairs, declaring proudly to his Granny and Grandpa that he had never felt so well in his life.

At a little after four thirty, I spotted the car outside the house, indicating to come onto the drive. Sitting in the passenger seat, with his blue Sick Children's Trust t-shirt on, was little Maxy. His face was illuminated with the biggest smile, and even from inside the house, you could see the look of unbridled excitement radiating from all his features. For nearly one ninth of his life, he had been away from that most important place, that place that 'makes no show to move'; home. It speaks of unconditional love, safety and security – so important for a little boy, who too soon in his life had been cast onto the cruel and unforgiving ocean.

Harry had made his way upstairs and was pretending to be unaware of Max's return, so that his brother could surprise him. As Max walked into the conservatory at the back of the house, he saw the banner above the door into the snug and he turned and gave me a massive hug. "Thanks, Dad," he said. We then launched into the mentally well-rehearsed plan. Whilst Max lingered in each room for a polite amount of time – almost out of a sense of duty to honour the homecoming blueprint – it was clear that he was itching to get to the main event; his bedroom.

Downstairs rooms all ticked off the list, with some excellent powers of memory and observation by Max in relation to minor changes, we climbed the stairs. Firstly, into the bathroom at the top, where I had toiled over the fitting of a thermostatic power shower – what a nightmare that had been, with more leaks than a government department in revolt, but I'd got there in the end. Then his brother's room, where Harry was seated in his little study-cum-cubby hole, ready to feign surprise at Max's appearance. Joke delivered, the brothers stood and embraced for what seemed like an age – this was confirmation, if any were needed, of just how much these two boys loved one another. Harry had lived with the spectre of Max never coming home to him, and although life would never be quite the same again, he was holding his little, warm, properly perfuse and very happy younger brother in his arms. As a boy of a similar age to Harry, I had encountered my first experience of bereavement; my Great Auntie, Jinny, who had spoiled me rotten with sweets and pocket money. How I had cried, when this lovely eighty-four-year-old had died. How on earth then, must Harry have felt for all of this time, knowing that there was a very real chance he would lose his brother? Harry is a bright kid – he understood the odds as well as we did. Well, he hadn't lost Max, and he now held the living, breathing proof of the wonder of life in his arms.

Embraces relinquished, Max made his way across the landing, eyes closed and under Harry's guidance, into his room. As he opened his eyes, he fell silent, just looking around his new kingdom with his mouth slightly ajar, drinking in the sight that greeted him. His beloved stereo, no longer on his bedside table, was now housed in a purpose-built rack, the speakers set up to deliver a correctly imaging stereo sound. Opposite was the huge reclining, swivelling listening chair, which had the added bonuses of being heated and massaging. Along one wall was his new bunk bed and a shelf, built into the chimney recess at bed height, which meant that he could have his beloved KEF speakers with him as he slept. A lucky little boy? Yes, you bet, but after the experience he had been through and taking into account the challenges to come, he thoroughly deserved it. "It's epic…thank you so much." That's all I needed to hear.

We had a cuddle, and I said, "Welcome home, Maxy." We all shed a tear.

DIARY OF A HEART MUM: Thirtieth Weekly Update – Sunday, 27 August 2017.

So, it's been three weeks since my last update. In that time, we were transferred to the Scott House Transplant flat, which allowed us to adjust to life outside the ward, whilst still being near the hospital for clinic and bloods.

We ventured to a few places after 14:00 medication, such as Alnwick Castle and Gardens, Hadrian's Wall, the beach and Beamish outdoor museum, always being mindful about keeping away from groups of people.

Also feel comfortable and knowledgeable about the medication now. Lots of it, but should reduce.

Max loved the transplant flat and has been going from strength to strength. The operation has really transformed him and we are so grateful to have him, and that the donor family agreed. Max's new heart came just at the right time!

We were finally officially discharged on Thursday and we said our goodbyes, including a lovely meal at Norma's house on the Wednesday evening. Quite emotional after 245 days in hospital, 206 of those days spent waiting for a new heart!

Arrived home, and Max loved his new bedroom. It was wonderful to be back as a complete family after being so disjointed and fragmented for so long. I won't miss Wetherby Services! (Although, we have started travelling up the M6 to Carlisle and

180

*then across to Newcastle as there are fewer roadworks/delays).
Max's first request was a kid's meal at Subway, so we tootled
along before the lunch rush. Luckily, very quiet!*

*As I type this, Max and I are back in Newcastle, staying near
the hospital, ready for 8:30 clinic tomorrow morning, when he has
bloods taken, weight checked, ECHO, ECG, urine tests and
meeting with Dr Reinhardt and Terry, the transplant nurse
specialist, with whom Max always enjoys a joke and some banter.
I start back to work on Wednesday, so that will be strange.*

*Also, Max has been in the Mirror again recently, raising
awareness.*

*Allowing myself to start relaxing a bit, but will feel better once
we are through the first three months post-transplant and then
again the first year post-transplant.*

*I will do occasional updates as and when. Thanks to everyone
for the lovely comments of support over the last nine months, and
so sorry I haven't always managed a reply. They have been
appreciated. Love, Emma X.*

*"Thanks for all your updates, Em, over the last few very difficult
months. Your strength has been amazing. So thrilled that the
outcome for Max and you all has been so wonderful. Max seems to
be going from strength to strength, and long may it continue!
Thinking of you as always, and much love to you all from us all xx.
The Finnigans."*

*"That is all fantastic. Everyone is so happy that Max is home
and we appreciate all you have done to keep us so well informed.
Now you can afford to relax a little as a family and begin a renewed
life together again. Love to Max and Harry and to you and Paul who
have endured so much together. Well done! Malcolm and Sue xxx."*

I remember when Harry was born and we brought him home for
the first time, he had fallen asleep in the car. Carefully, so as not to
wake him, we'd carried him inside and placed him, still in his car
seat, on the rug in the front room. Emma and I had then looked at
one another and said, "What do we do now?" We hadn't got a clue
and the manual was blank. We now had similar feelings with Max
– no longer the veteran parents, the old sweats who knew what to
do – we were in similarly uncharted waters. We had some dinner –
well-cooked to minimise the risk of food poisoning – and sat and
looked at Max. He seemed okay, but our antennae were crackling

with awareness of our new situation and the need to be ready. What for, we didn't know, but we needed to be ready anyway!

Max returned home with a list of medications which had to be taken at 0800hrs, 1400hrs and 2000hrs. Those taken at 0800 and 2000 included his anti-rejection medication, which had to be administered to the strict timetable. At his weekly clinic visits, Max's blood would be checked for appropriate levels, and almost every week, his dosage would change. We became expert at dispensing various oily liquids from their bottles; it reminded me of chemistry lessons at school. Max preferred liquids at this time – in most cases, there was a choice between liquid and tablet form – as the tablets could (in the case of zeppelin-esque magnesium) be difficult to swallow. In fairness to Max, we were very lucky. He took his medication without fuss. At times in hospital, before his transplant, medication could make him sick, especially liquid Omeprazole. A protection for his tummy, the lining of which was disintegrating due to his poorly heart, the Omeprazole would illicit the gag reflex every time without fail. Bless him, he would be sick, but a quick rub of the back saw him barely break step with whatever he was doing. A brave little fella – some parents had a real battle with their children when it came to medication time – on this front, we were very lucky.

That first night in his own room was very special. Scott House, provided by The Sick Children's Trust, had the 'transplant flat'. A wonderfully equipped space with bedroom, bathroom and living room, it allowed children and parents who had become institutionalised over months at the hospital, to be together as a family again. It meant that you could begin the process of establishing the new norm for your lives, with the peace of mind in knowing that the ward was only a hike away along the Magnolia Mile.

Now at home, the process of establishing that new norm could enter its final phase. As bedtime approached, Max's medication was dispensed and placed into a blue plastic tray for him to consume. Warm, sweet milk was prepared to help it on its way. This done, Max's stereo system was powered-up and Sam Smith was placed onto his recently refurbished Bang and Olufsen Beogram 1203 turntable. This piece of classic audio equipment had belonged to my father, and as a child, I had been mesmerised by the smooth automatic mechanism and the sleek looks. After some forty years of faithful service, the turntable was given to Max, but it was in need of some tender loving care. As another project to occupy his mind during his long wait, I had found a chap who was able to service the motor and mechanism for me, whilst Max and I sat in the playroom garden and polished the wooden surround and cleaned the brushed aluminium top plate. It looked a million dollars, and as the stylus landed in the groove, we were enveloped by that wonderful sound that only vinyl can produce through some classic KEF speakers.

Max and I had listened to the Sam Smith album before he fell ill, alongside Lukas Graham's most recent release. As I sat in his big, reclining/swivelling/rocking chair with Max curled up in front of me on the capacious seat, I contemplated the journey we had been on and just how special this was. For months, we had talked of this moment – the 'listening sesh' we'd have – without knowing when, or if, it would ever happen. Well, thanks to an amazing chain of events and some hugely gifted and considerate people, here we now were. I gently stroked Max's soft cheek as he rested his head and closed his eyes and I drank the moment in. To be sitting with my beautiful little boy like this was all that I had wanted, all that I had prayed for and now my prayers had been answered. Sam Smith never sounded so good.

In hospital, Max had a disco light set up, which filled his bed space with all of the colours of the rainbow at night. Now, this light was placed on the floor in his room, positioned in such a way that the light array filled his kingdom with tiny, orbiting planets of light, which traced a consistent path across his walls and ceiling. Sitting in Max's chair next to his bed – as I had done night after night in hospital – I looked at these lights, with increasingly distant, smudged vision, whilst Max slowly relented his grip on the world of 'busy awake' and dropped to sleep. Due to the potency of some of his medicines, immediate sleep was not a given and the whole bedtime routine took an inordinately long time to complete. I'm not complaining – it is a small price to pay – so what if my presence is required, invariably in pensive mood, as Max tries to get to sleep; I'd only be sitting with my body and mind in neutral in front of the television.

Sometimes in an evening and as a consequence of the powerful medication he is required to take, Max would complain of a headache. As a transplanted patient, he had to avoid ibuprofen, so painkillers of the paracetamol kind would be administered. Frequently, Max was clearly poleaxed by these headaches; he would curl up into the foetal position on a chair and go very quiet; his distress was present to see. It is to be expected that medication that

183

does such drastic things to your body, is going to come with a sting in the tail. Other side effects also presented.

Immediately post-transplant, Max was placed onto an anti-rejection drug called Cyclosporin. This is the drug of choice, not least because it can be administered intravenously and this allows for easier tweaking. Taken for long enough, Cyclosporin causes hair to grow in places where before smoothness had prevailed. Now, on a hairy, post-pubescent male of the species, this would probably not be too much of an issue. However, on a pre-pubescent light blonde little man, the effects are more, shall we say, transformational. Max grew a soft down all over his body, and his eyebrows – before a faint hint – were now Dennis Healey incarnate. The pictures taken by the Daily Mirror in Max's bedroom, soon after his return home, show how his eyebrows had become darker and thicker. To his credit, this did not really bother Max, who actually became quite fond of his down. At the right moment in time, doctors transferred Max onto a new anti-rejection drug called Tacrolimus, the bonus being that his furry coat gradually washed down the plughole and the shade of his eyebrows lightened by a tint or two.

At the end of September 2017, Emma was invited to the Labour Party Conference in Brighton and she was a guest speaker at one of the fringe events organised by the Mirror to try and promote the Mirror campaign. Emma had never attended a political conference before and wasn't sure what to expect. She was concerned that, if interviewed, she might be treated like a politician, in a combative fashion. Really, she was just an ordinary mum whose son had suffered some extraordinary misfortune. This had led to Emma's determination and passion that something needed to be done about the organ donation rules. When you watch your child suffering, languishing on a 'waiting list' and you know that thousands of others across the country, adult and child, are doing the same, then this springboard that starts with compassion can very quickly evolve into a single-minded resolve to 'do something'. Sitting on the train, Emma wanted to feel prepared so she did a lot of background reading around the subject. She was well looked after at the conference and there was no hostile interviewing as she had feared. Emma managed not to be daunted by other panel members, who all had their own powerful and inspiring stories to tell. She even managed to enjoy a couple of cocktails on the sea front and blew out some cobwebs.

Although petrified, Emma decided that the bigger picture was too important to let her 'smaller' insecurities get in the way. This is her speech:

"Our nine-year-old son Max was a normal, healthy, fun-loving child – then on December 8th last year, he was rushed to hospital, and it was found that he had an enlarged heart. He was suffering from heart failure.

He spent a night at Leighton Hospital in Crewe and after his condition deteriorated, the team there acted quickly to stabilise him and arrange a safe, urgent transfer to the Royal Manchester Children's Hospital. There, he was diagnosed with a condition called dilated cardiomyopathy. His heart had become so large that it was no longer able to pump the blood around his body effectively. We were told that our son had a 33% chance of getting better, a 33% chance of requiring a heart transplant and a 33% chance of passing away. Our world was turned upside down.

Max soldiered on under the superb care in Manchester, but he was not getting any better, and in early January, he was transferred to the Freeman Hospital in Newcastle-upon-Tyne, where he was assessed and placed on the urgent list for a heart transplant! The wait had begun.

Max's condition continued to deteriorate, and so in early February, he had open-heart surgery to fit a mechanical pump to assist his own heart function. We were bowled over by the availability of such intricate technology and by the skill, dedication and compassion that we witnessed in all three hospitals.

We knew that Max could not stay like this indefinitely and that he desperately needed a new heart, but Max's positive attitude, courage and wit saw him through numerous ups and downs in his condition.

The hardest part of waiting for a compatible organ was the not knowing when or if one would become available, and whether Max would be able to stay stable enough for long enough to withstand such a serious operation.

After over six months waiting, the call finally came in August, and Max was successfully transplanted. We will forever be indebted to a family out there that made the courageous decision to say 'yes' to organ donation at such a devastating time.

We have gained an incredible insight into the work of this unique and truly wonderful NHS facility at the Freeman Hospital. The sheer number of specialists involved in the care of one little boy, and how they all work together to make important, well considered and caring decisions is quite remarkable. We are so grateful to the wonderful Dr Reinhardt, the incredible, yet humble Mr Hasan and his surgical team, to the nurses, sisters, doctors, cardiologists, transplant teams, psychologists, play specialists, and not forgetting, the lovely Barbara, who kept Max's bed space spick and span. The list goes on! These people were the silver lining around our cloud and helped to keep Max motivated and comfortable during his ordeal. Newcastle is indeed very close to our hearts and we will miss the Geordie cappuccinos, complete with 'chocolate sprinkles' (said in Geordie). Try saying Betablockers in Geordie!

On a serious note, Max has been lucky and is going from strength to strength in his recovery and is starting to pick up the pieces of his old life. Others are not so lucky!

It is so important to recognise that there are over 6000 people in England currently waiting for a lifesaving organ transplant. For some of those people, the wait will be too long, and they will pass away or become too ill before they are given the chance of a new life. Last year, 470 people, including 14 children, died whilst on the transplant list or died after they had been taken off the list because they had become too ill for surgery. Ironically, in the same period, 460 organs suitable for transplant were not used because of lack of consent. Permission is refused by family members of suitable donors because consent was not actively given in advance through the Organ Donor Register. Without that consent, families often understandably hesitate and the window of opportunity is lost.

Reporter Jeremy Armstrong and the Mirror newspaper have campaigned to 'Change the Law for Life', in conjunction with MPs – Geoffrey Robinson and Dan Jarvis debating and putting forward the 'Organ Donation Deemed Consent Bill' – affectionately dubbed 'Max's Law!'. If we change the law to one of 'opt out', everyone is considered to consent to organ donation, unless they declare otherwise.

The second reading of the bill is on the 23 February 2018. In the meantime, if you haven't already done so, please consider registering on the Organ Donor Register and most importantly, discuss your wishes with your family. In England, we find it easy to arrange life insurance and to write wills, but we don't always discuss what we want to happen with our own bodies when we die. Let's break the taboo and have the conversation! I would like to finish by emphasising that what has happened to Max and our family could happen to anyone. This time last year, we had no idea what was about to hit us. Statistically, we are more likely to require a lifesaving transplant than we are to ever become an organ donor. Therefore, when it comes to the vote, I ask you to consider all those patients of all ages waiting desperately for the 'gift of life' and I urge you to 'opt in' to saving lives and 'opt out' to standing by and doing nothing."

DIARY OF A HEART MUM: Thirty-First Weekly Update (The last one!) Sunday, 15 October 2017.

So, Max has been home just over four weeks. He is doing very well and is loving life. Private tuition two hours a day for three days a week has started, and he is really trying hard. Luckily, his teacher was his teacher at school in Year 1 and 2, so they know each other well.

Clinics have been going well and his new heart is consistently described as 'happy' and 'brilliant'. Max is adjusting to all the medication, and he now has beautiful bushy eyebrows and a lovely furry back, but it is blonde so really not noticeable. We are still in the 'infection-risk' zone, or 'quarantine', as we call it. But friends and family have been very understanding about the fact that Max can't mingle with more than one or two occasional visitors. Max will have his immunology bloods taken tomorrow morning, which will give us an idea about when he can mingle/start school etc. Fingers crossed. We will still be very conscious of infection risk though, whatever the decision.

Other news, the 'Change the Law for Life' organ donation campaign continued at full throttle, and I was very brave, delivering a speech at the Labour Party Conference about Max's story. They played a video with Max being interviewed and I really had to hold it together! The other speakers were outstanding!

Then a week after the conference, Theresa May announced, out of the blue, that she would be changing the law on organ donation! Just amazing and very unexpected. A few days later, a letter dropped through our door. It was from Theresa May to Max, explaining that Max's story had inspired her to change the law and that she and her government would be calling it 'Max's Law'. Just incredible, and we are so proud of Max. That boy done good. What a turnaround, from something so negative to something so positive!

So exciting! We have quite a few thank you letters to write.

On other news, I went back to work four weeks ago and have been enjoying the role. Really varied and I'm so much more relaxed at work, and I don't think this has gone unnoticed. Starting to joke around a bit and enjoy the banter, which was hard whilst Max was in hospital.

Thank you all again for your wonderful support and encouragement. Love, Em X.

"Hi, Emma. So lovely to read such positive news after all the trauma. Much hope now for a brighter future for you all. Much love, Nic xx."

On one visit to clinic in the winter of 2017, Max and Emma stayed with Geordie guardian angel, Norma, and she took them for a walk in the snow to where everyone was sledging. Using her compelling powers of persuasion, Norma managed to convince a man to let Max have a go with his sledge. Max simply loved it – he revelled in the exhilaration and abandon of hurtling down the slope. Norma is so life-loving and young at heart – she got it. In many ways, Max and Norma are very similar in their outlook on life and I know that she will be our friend forever. Thank you, Norma, for all you did for our family when we were at our lowest.

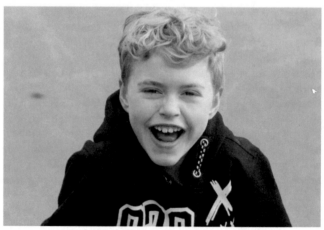

Max on one of his clinic visits to Newcastle
Photo Credit: Andy Commins/Mirror Newspaper Group

Just because Max now had the heart that he so desperately needed did not mean that the Mirror campaign was over. There were many more children and adults still playing 'the waiting game'. We were continuing to try so hard to raise awareness and increase consent rates. We wanted the public to understand the huge gratitude we felt towards our donor family (anonymous at this time) and donor families in general. By expressing that gratitude, it might encourage other bereaved families to consent to organ donation. The articles continued in August, September and October:

"'It's the best I've felt my whole life": Brave Max, nine, tells of delight after lifesaving heart transplant.'

'Heart transplant hero, Max Johnson, who languished on waiting list for eight months says 'biggest thank you' to donor.'

"'I'm happy to be home, but my friend wasn't so lucky": Heart swap hero Max repeats call for donor law change.'

'Mum of heart transplant hero, Max, pleads for help for the children on 'death row' waiting for new organs.'

It was in early October 2017 that Max received a letter from Prime Minister Theresa May. Initially, he had thought the letter was some sort of voucher. He handed me the envelope and I removed the thick sheet of paper from within. Immediately, my eyes were drawn to the header, which told me – straight away – where the correspondence was from. I nearly fell off that rocking, swivelling chair of Max's when I saw the signature! I said to Max: "This is not a voucher, Max, it's from the Prime Minister!" He was awestruck when he saw the '10 Downing Street' header at the top of the letter, which said:

"Dear Max,

I hope you are feeling much better after your heart transplant and are enjoying being back home with your Mum and Dad.

I wanted to write to you after hearing about your bravery.

When I read your inspirational story, I knew I had to change the organ donation rules to an 'opt out' system. Your parents must be so proud of what you have achieved – with much more still to come, I'm sure.

I also read that you thought it would be fun to name the change in the rules after you.

I think that's a brilliant idea – so whilst it will have to have a bit of a boring title when it goes through Parliament – I and my government will call it 'Max's Law'.

Can I end by saying how pleased I am that the NHS was able to help you and hundreds of people just like you?

Our doctors, nurses and NHS staff do amazing things every day and – once the law is changed – I hope even more transplants will be able to take place and more lives will be saved.

With Best Wishes,
Theresa May."

The headline soon followed:

'Donor law will be called 'Max's Law' in honour of little boy whose bravery helped change Britain.'

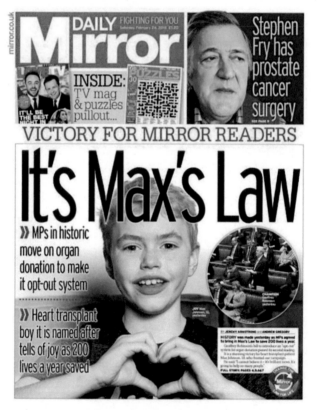

Max on the Mirror front cover
Photo Credit: Andy Stenning/Mirror Newspaper Group

We were hugely reassured that Max and the Mirror's Change the Law for Life campaign had the support of so many eminent professionals and organisations, such as the British Medical Association (who had been campaigning for this law change for many years), Kidney Care UK, the Royal College of Physicians, the British Heart Foundation and pioneering heart surgeons, Sir Terence English and Sir Magdi Yacoub. Mr Asif Hasan, paediatric transplant surgeon and Director of Heart and Lung Transplantation at Newcastle's Freeman Hospital said:

"Nearly 20% of patients – adults and children – die whilst waiting for an organ to become available. We are extremely grateful to all relatives and donor families as the donation of an organ is vital to saving hundreds of lives. Yet we still need to do more. We're proud to support this lifesaving appeal and it's really easy for everyone to take part – just have a chat. That chat might be the next time you sit down for a meal, when you are shopping or working, or just driving in the car."

We were very much in awe of the incredible Mr Hasan and anytime we had bumped into him in the hospital corridor, we always had to control our urge to bow down and pay homage! So, we were delighted when, in December 2017, Max and Emma were able to spend some time with Mr Hasan at the Science Museum in London. They had been invited to the 50th Anniversary celebration (organised by the Papworth Hospital team) of the first ever heart transplant which took place in South Africa, performed by Christiaan Barnard. Max was to be a guest speaker amongst a crowd of wonderful heart surgeons and staff, including pioneering heart surgeon, Sir Terence English. Max delivered a PowerPoint presentation, 'My Heart Story', with aplomb. Emma was so proud of him standing up there in his electric blue suit and matching 'Heelys'! How far he had come! Max and Mr Hasan shared some nice chats together and had some pictures taken with one another. There was a heart-shaped cake, which Max got to cut – with a scalpel! The Mirror was there to follow Max's ongoing journey.

'Amazing moment transplant boy, Max Johnson, meets the hero surgeon who saved his life.'

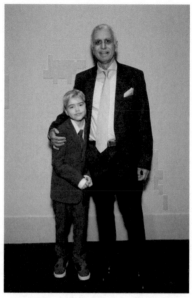

Max with his heart surgeon, Mr Asif Hasan
Photo Credit: Mirror Newspaper Group

It was always a surprise to us how dramatic and impactful the headlines of the Mirror articles were, and we would sometimes blink and find it hard to comprehend that the subject matter was our own son and family. Now that Max was home, we were starting to see so much good coming out of a situation that had been so horrific. The Mirror had very much taken Max under their media 'wing' ('Our Max' and 'Mirror Boy Max'), and there seemed to be a public fascination with this little fellow's progress. Even his return to school was detailed in a Mirror article:

'Heart swap hero, Max Johnson, is back at school – and he spent first day back raising money for Children in Need.'

Whilst Max was beginning to readjust to life at home, his bravery was starting to be recognised, winning a Commendation Certificate in the WellChild Awards, a Your Champions 'Young Person of the Year' award, presented by athlete, Colin Jackson, and a 'Young Person of the Year' award at Winsford's very own 'Town

Mayor's Oscars'! Crikey, we had to be careful this didn't all go to Max's head!

Max also agreed to appear several times on BBC North West Tonight as the media followed the progress of the law. It just so happens that my brother and Max's Uncle, Roger, is the presenter on this show, so we felt very relaxed about being involved. My brother, his wife, Lucy, and their three boys, James, Edward and William, had been fantastic whilst Max was ill, visiting Newcastle on a number of occasions and offering help and practical support where they could. So, it was lovely to be interviewed by such a trusted family member, without the usual 'media' nerves!

Other appearances included BBC Radio Five Live, CBBC Newsround and social media videos for NHS Blood & Transplant and the British Heart Foundation. Max wanted to encourage people to register on the Organ Donor Register and also to give blood; just as lifesaving as organ donation. Max and our family were so happy to support the British Heart Foundation as they had set aside ten million pounds to research dilated cardiomyopathy and they are conducting important research into lengthening the lives of heart patients post-transplant. (20% of heart transplant patients die within ten years of their operation. A sobering statistic!)

One of the highest profile and national broadcasts that Max was involved with, was the BBC 2 Documentary 'Heart Transplant – A Chance to Live', which aired in May 2018. Along with six other brave patients, the programme followed Max's journey from before the transplant, it filmed his actual transplant and featured a post-operation interview some weeks later. This beautifully crafted piece of documentary work resulted in an increase of 588% in people registering to be organ donors. It was described as 'the best advertisement for organ donation'.

It was very poignant watching this. Seeing your son lying on the operating table without a heart, as the bypass machine kept him alive, is a moment I will never forget. The contrast of Max's huge, scarred old heart with that beautiful, petite new heart was striking. How on earth had Max managed to survive with such congestion! This was also the moment that we saw the incredible skill of the surgical team in stemming a difficult, sudden and unexpected bleed. The documentary really drummed home just how poorly Max had been with Mr Hasan, in his pre-transplant interview, declaring sadly, "Max was in imminent danger of death. We thought his heart would stop at any time."

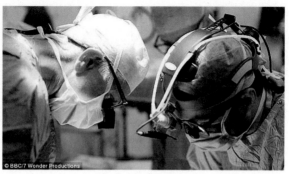

Heart surgeons, Mr Asif Hasan and Mr Fabrizio de Rita during Max's heart transplant.
Photo Credit: Heart Transplant – A Chance to Live. Director James W. Newton. 7Wonder Productions/BBC Two

What moved us to tears was seeing how frightened Max was before he was put to sleep for the operation and those haunting words, "I love you both!" The documentary ended with Max dancing and squealing with delight in the pouring rain. What a message! Enjoy every moment life gives you and appreciate the small things. *Everyone should have a chance to dance in the rain!* These images seemed to sum up the generosity of organ donation and the 'gift of life' that results from 'saying yes'. Max's snippets on the documentary were also shown on Channel Four's Gogglebox the following Friday. We found that very touching to watch, as we could see the sympathy of ordinary people viewing Max's story for the first time, but it was also very uplifting to hear the outpouring of love for our wonderful NHS.

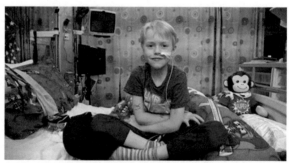

Max in 'Heart Transplant: A Chance to Live'
Photo Credit: Heart Transplant: A Chance to Live. Director James W. Newton. 7Wonder Productions/BBC Two

In August 2018, the government announced that the new law would be implemented in 2020 and as with all such announcements, it was covered across the media, triggering debate and discussion. Max and Emma agreed to be interviewed by Paddy O'Connell on Radio 4's Sunday morning show, Broadcasting House. It was a great experience and they were able to share our thoughts about the benefits a law change might bring. It was also amusing to hear Paddy O'Connell's trepidation before speaking with Max. What do they say about children and animals? As with any law change, there were always going to be people who were opposed. (NB: a minority voice, as the vast majority of the record 17,000 people/organisations who responded to the government consultation, were in favour of the changes). We didn't mind that there would be people who may wish to 'opt out' for personal or religious reasons. What troubled us were those who protested that the 'opt out' proposals were 'bodysnatching' or 'the government *taking* your organs'. It would not be 'forced donation' – the law change would mean that everybody would automatically be considered to be an organ donor, unless they had chosen to opt out. Furthermore, the family would still have the final say. People would just need to make their wishes known to their family and…hopefully… their family would say 'yes' or 'no' accordingly. Organ donation would remain a precious gift. If people didn't agree with organ donation, they could just 'opt out'. It would still be a choice. It would be very simple and clear to 'opt out' if they so wished.

I was reminded of an interview I'd heard with a transplant surgeon from Bristol. Max had appeared on the same broadcast, but the words of this surgeon really hit home. One evening, he had tucked his little daughter into bed before leaving for work. She had been wearing her favourite 'Paw Patrol' pyjamas – she was a huge fan of this children's cartoon. Her father's role that night was to recover some precious gifts from a donor, whose family had made the courageous decision to say 'yes' to organ donation. As he entered the theatre, he caught his first sight of the donor; a precious four-year-old boy, who was wearing the exact same 'Paw Patrol' pyjamas as his daughter. The surgeon recounted that there was not a dry eye in the operating theatre that night. Our experience of transplantation holds true to the picture, so movingly painted by this recollection. People who we encountered during our time in Newcastle, charged with managing and delivering transplant surgery were compassionate to the very nucleus of their being; nobody understood, nor appreciated more, the hugely powerful emotions which engulfed and wrapped donor families, recipients and their loved ones.

The goal of the law change would be to increase the consent rate by propagating family conversations, through the scale of publicity that would happen throughout 2019, to prepare people for the changes. Many forget that they may benefit from this change in legislation one day, if they or a member of their family end up requiring a lifesaving organ. 'Soft opt out' in other countries (over twenty countries in Europe alone) has led to increased family conversations, more 'known decisions', an increased consent rate, shorter hospital waits for organs, and fewer people dying waiting for an eligible organ. It is a springboard or catalyst for encouraging organ donation to be part of the public consciousness rather than a taboo topic. The new law should trigger improved education and campaigns, a change in cultural mindset and a strengthening of the infrastructure and transplant co-ordinator capacity. England has the lowest consent rate in Europe and this law change might just help to transform that. We were also very aware that, although a sizeable 38% of people were signed up on the Organ Donor Register, roughly 80% supported organ donation and wouldn't mind donating, but many never got around to signing up or telling their family. We felt that a change to a 'soft opt out' system might help to address this and increase the pool of organ donors. At least, we thought, let's give it a go.

Dave Nicholson's post-transplant interview with Max at Radio Tyneside was given a Gold award for 'Best Speech Package' at the HBA National Radio Awards. What was so touching is that Dave surprised Max at clinic one day and presented him with the award. Max had finished the interview by saying, "If anyone is waiting in hospital, please don't give up. That gift will come eventually." He knew just how they felt.

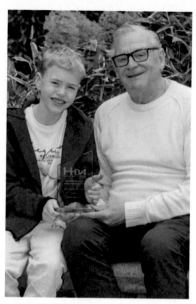

Dave Nicholson of Radio Tyneside presents Max with the HBA award
Photo Credit: Andy Commins/Mirror Newspaper Group

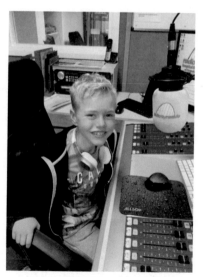

Max in Radio Tyneside Studios
Photo Credit: Dave Nicholson

Our media involvement may seem like a lot to take on board, but these appearances didn't take too much of our time, and we were able to try and get some semblance of balance back in our lives. We derived great pleasure from doing the seemingly 'normal' and mundane activities that we had so missed when Max had fallen ill; walks to the shops, tennis games, trips to McDonald's, going swimming, playing in the park and walks along Whitegate Way. Occasionally, Max's memories of a very difficult journey would catch up with him, and he would break down in tears. It was often music that triggered these meltdowns. 'In My Blood' by Shawn Mendes was one such song. Some of the lyrics reminded him of how trapped he had often felt in hospital.

So, is it worth it? Well, I am typing this overlooking a beautiful, if slightly overcast scene straight out of one of Alfred Wainwright's books on the Lake District, in a small village called Ireby. Sitting six feet away from me is Max, watching videos on YouTube. Yesterday, we went for a long walk over the hill behind the cottage and it was only the inclement weather which stopped Max from launching a serious assault on Binsey Hill, such were his energy levels and sheer zest for life and adventure. Binsey Hill might as well be the north face of the Eiger for me, so to climb it would be an achievement for all of us. To sit at the dining table and to see Max's cheeky grin and be on the receiving end of his wicked sense of humour is indubitably reward enough for all of the hardships we have endured and will endure as a family, and is a testament to the brilliance of the Freeman Hospital and the selfless humanity of our donor family. You just have to accept that life is more about the here and now, one day at a time. I'll say it again; Carpe Diem.

All paediatric transplant recipients at the Freeman are referred to an incredible charity called 'Make-A-Wish'. It is an acknowledgement that transplantation, however remarkable, is life limiting. For his 'wish', Max decided to indulge his love of speakers and sound by requesting a trip to the KEF Loudspeaker factory, which is based in Kent.

Having met with our local 'Make-A-Wish' facilitators, who came to the house to discuss the wish with Max, a date was set for us to visit KEF. In July 2018, we made the trip to London, where we were put up in a hotel next to the London Eye. Every detail – and I mean every detail – had been thought through. Not only were train tickets provided, we were collected from the station by a taxi and taken to our hotel. From that point on and until we returned home two days later, we were transported everywhere in a stretch limousine! Our wish coincided with the visit to the UK of the United States President, Donald J. Trump. His presence had attracted a fair degree of protest in London, so as we sat in the inevitable traffic jams around the centre of our capital, our limousine was cast asunder by some thunderous looks. I am sure that, had the protestors realised that the occupant, far from being public enemy number one President Trump, was in fact a little boy on his 'Make-A-Wish' treat, they'd have softened their demeanour!

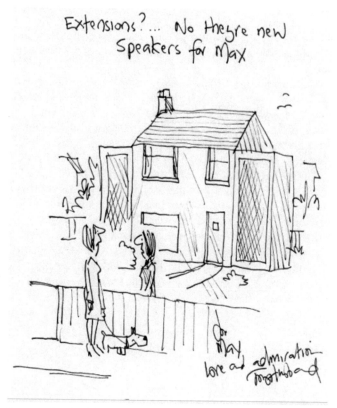

Cartoon sketched for Max by Private Eye Cartoonist – Tony Husband

Our visit to the KEF factory was very special indeed, in no small measure due to the warmth and kindness of our hosts, who must have been somewhat bemused by this ever-so-slightly left field request. A visit to the anechoic chamber, the computer design lab and the production line, where Max got to play with a subwoofer, which literally rattled the rafters of the cavernous factory, made for a fascinating and different experience. We finished in the main listening room, which adjoins the KEF loudspeaker museum. Hidden under what I can only describe as sheets, were the monolithic Muons; KEF's sculptural flagship, limited edition speaker, affordable only to Captains of Industry and Premier League footballers. You know the adage; if you have to ask how much…

The sound, powered by some pristine, high-end Accuphase amplification was as you would expect it to be from a pair of loudspeakers costing as much as a house. However, what was really touching was that the music we were treated to came from Max's personal playlist and it had never – and I mean never – sounded so good.

We said goodbye to the wonderful team at KEF, who had really pulled the stops out for us, and headed back into London. That evening, and again thanks to 'Make-A-Wish', we went to see Matilda the Musical. What a generous, thoughtful and beautifully choreographed experience – yet again, a charity making all the difference.

Another key turning point for Max was taking part in the school sports day in the summer term of 2018; unthinkable the year before as he lay in his hospital bed. Emma wrote on Facebook: "Max's lovely new heart powered him to victory in the Sports Day sprint…what a milestone and a fitting metaphor for winning his battle against heart failure. Visited by a little robin too as Max crossed the finish line. Thank you, Keira! Life after transplant."

You may well wonder who Keira is. Well, all will be explained…

Chapter 13

'"Keira's heart could not wait to start beating inside him": Incredible moment transplant boy Max gets new heart'

This was the Mirror headline, following the airing of the BBC 2 Documentary 'Heart Transplant: A Chance to Live' in May, 2018, which showed Max's life-saving heart transplant. Keira Ball was Max's organ donor, a little girl, aged nine. But how did we learn about this treasured child?

"Hello, I'm Loanna… I'd like to thank you so much for your cards and so pleased to see Max is doing so well. We would love to keep in touch and I'd like to say Max has got the most beautiful heart in the world."

These gentle words appeared innocuously as a private message out of the blue in Emma's Facebook account on 20 October 2017. We were getting ready to go away for a week, our first holiday since Max came home. Emma had decided to quickly check Facebook for any messages before setting off. A few weeks beforehand, Emma had bumped into Alison, our Transplant Coordinator, at Max's regular clinic. Emma had asked whether there was any information available about Max's donor. Alison showed Emma and Max into a private room and shared with them, in the usual sensitive and kind fashion, that Max's donor had been a nine-year-old girl.

Max went quiet as he listened and Emma shed a tear; the suffocating sadness that the donor family must be experiencing and the heartbreak for the donor herself became all the more imaginable and real. Until that point, everything felt somewhat vague and abstract. A heart had become available and Max had a 'second chance', but we knew nothing about the donor, except for a hint that the heart was 'age appropriate'.

Emma thanked Alison and asked whether we could write thank you cards. Alison said yes, and that cards could be passed to her and she would then arrange for them to be forwarded to the donor family. We could put our first names, but no other details such as surnames or address, were allowed. Our knowledge that the donor was a nine-year-old girl, had somehow given a sense of urgency, of gravitas, to the need to express our gratitude to the donor family. So, we set about writing a card. This was so difficult to compose. How on earth do you begin to thank someone, whose decision has effectively saved your son's life and given him the chance of a future? Would we be able to find appropriate words that captured how indebted we felt? Emma and I sat down and spent a good few hours writing our thoughts. This is what we came up with:

"To Max's donor family,

We are writing to you as you hold a very special place in our hearts. Our son, Max, is nine and he had a heart transplant on 2nd August.

He was very poorly and a heart transplant was his only chance of coming home and starting a new life.

We are so sorry that you lost your beloved child, but we would like to thank you for the incredibly kind, courageous decision that you made to allow your child's organs to be donated. We do not know the circumstances, but we can only imagine what a dreadful, harrowing time you have been through and are doubtless still going through, with the loss of your precious child.

Even in your grief, you have made a selfless decision to help others and we are indescribably grateful to you.

We hope that it brings you some comfort to know that Max's post-transplant recovery has been smooth and without complication. His new heart has been described as a 'happy heart' and a 'brilliant heart'. Max is very thankful and he is looking after his new heart. He says 'Good Morning' to his new heart every day and sends it lots of love, whilst it adjusts to the new environment. He is eating healthily and exercising when he feels able, so that his heart will stay fit and strong.

Max is getting used to all the medication, but he is full of energy and enthusiasm, as a result of the new lease of life that has been gifted by your family. He is relishing every moment back at home, without sickness, tubes, wires, machines, procedures etc. It was a very upsetting time, waiting so long for the call, but when we did get the call, we prayed for you and your family. We continue to pray for you and think about you.

We wanted you to know that your child's passing was not in vain and your child has an incredible legacy of love and goodwill to others.

We thank you so much for making a decision that has saved our son and given him the prospect of a future ahead of him. As he grows older, we will encourage him to cherish his heart in memory of your child.

With all our love and eternal gratitude,

Emma and Paul."

We also had a strong urge that we wanted our donor family to know who Max was and what a difference their decision had made to a young boy's life. So, we took the difficult decision to share our letter with the Mirror Newspaper for two reasons: firstly, we thought that this would enable the donor family to reach out to us. Emma felt that if she tried to put herself in the donor family's shoes, then knowing a little bit about the child you had saved could bring a small measure of comfort. By this time, we had realised the power of the media and the positive effects the Mirror campaign was having in terms of raising awareness about organ donation. Secondly, we believed that by publicising our gratitude, it would help people to see the difference that organ donation makes and might therefore encourage them to sign up on the Organ Donor Register, hopefully increasing the consent rate amongst bereaved families.

Sure enough, our incredible donor family put two and two together and identified that Max was the recipient of their beautiful daughter's heart, although one of their family members had wondered earlier whether this might be the case.

So, on 20 October 2017, as we sat in the conservatory getting ready to go away, and Emma opened her laptop, I was shocked when she suddenly broke down in tears. "What's the matter?" I asked. Emma couldn't reply, as she was overcome with emotion. Once she had recovered, she read to me the message from Loanna. I was so moved; we felt as though we had somehow come full circle and that the final piece of the organ donation jigsaw had slotted into place.

As Emma and Loanna continued to share messages, a very special and rare bond was formed. She explained to Emma what had happened that fateful day on 30th July 2017. Loanna, Bradley (aged seven) and Keira (aged nine) had been involved in a terrible, tragic car crash. Loanna and Bradley were seriously injured and Keira died from her injuries. Our hero, Joe Ball, Keira's father, in such unimaginable, heartrending circumstances, with his wife and son in different hospitals, made the decision to donate Keira's organs. His brave act saw four people receive a lifesaving gift in the opening days of August 2017.

To us and everybody that knows this story, it was an incredible act of kindness, selflessness and humanity. It is impossible to comprehend how Joe must have been feeling – his own heart shattered, he did something indescribably beautiful.

As we have gradually got to know the Ball family, including their other two daughters and son, Keely-Rose, Katelyn and Bradley, we feel a very special connection to them; two families at different ends of the country thrown together by fate. Two sides of the organ donation coin – one the donor, and the other the recipient.

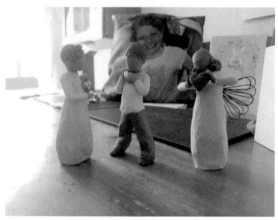

Willow Tree Figurines, with Keira's photo in the background
Photo Credit: Joe Ball

The more we learn about this beautiful little girl, Keira, the more we feel that she is truly a part of our family and forever will be – forever nine, forever giving. We have gained a spiritual daughter who we think of every day. Whilst we grieve for Keira, we also know that without Joe's decision, our son Max might not be here. There we have it – such conflicting emotions – how can they possibly co-exist? This could be why our brains sometimes feel foggy and we are emotionally all at sea. No one would ever wish for such a tragic accident to have happened, but the love and kindness of Keira and her family saved Max's life. We rejoice for Max, but we mourn for Keira and her family. In the midst of their grief, the Ball family continued to think of others, as they set up a charity called 'InspiredbyKeira', which encourages organ donation and also helps bereaved families who have lost children; such courage in terrible adversity.

So, we had established contact with a very special family, but we were yet to meet.

Organ donation, for all concerned, is an intensely personal and moving experience. Such are the immense, all-consuming emotions involved, that a decision to contact – let alone meet – needs careful consideration and has to be right for all parties. It is rare for recipients to meet the families of donors; great care is exercised by transplant co-ordinators to prevent people being put into difficult, emotionally damaging situations. Festina Lente: 'make haste slowly'. Our relationship with Joe and Loanna grew organically, starting with Loanna's beautiful message of introduction. Emma and I, once we had reflected on Loanna's courageous contact, had resolved that we would take things at a pace to suit the Ball family. We had our little boy and it didn't take much imagination to appreciate that meeting Max for the first time could be difficult for them.

For the entire week of our holiday, Emma would check her Facebook account for further contact. Facebook 'friends' requests were accepted as a starter for ten, then the exchange of photographs, where we got to look into the smiling, twinkling eyes of Max's donor, Keira, for the first time. It is a unique, affecting experience, to look at the face of someone you know has died, and yet their very essence, their very core, beats on in the chest of your son. It was incredible to think that only six months separated Max and Keira's birth, with Max being the first to declare his arrival in the world. To see the images of this captivating little girl – either a sparkling smile to the camera – or in action on her beloved pony, brought home the enormity of her loss. A little girl, only a few hundred yards into her journey of ten thousand miles, with a life stretching out before her, now gone well before her time. A life of hopes and dreams forever paused at the tender age of nine. How humbled, then, were we that Joe Ball had decided to make a gift of something so incredibly precious, so that Max's life could be given a chance to resume and flourish. This is how, with Keira's family's blessing, Emma introduced this gorgeous child, to her friends on Facebook:

"So, today is a milestone for Max, as it is 12 weeks to the day since his heart transplant on 2nd August. Max's donor family received our thank you cards recently and have reached out and made contact with us. They are truly lovely, amazing and incredibly brave. With their blessing, I would like to introduce a very special little girl called Keira. Keira lost her life in sudden and tragic circumstances. Max received this precious child's heart soon after.

Keira was only nine years old, but she will always be remembered and will live on in our family. At clinic appointments, Max's new heart has been invariably described with adjectives such as 'happy' and 'brilliant'. Looking at this lovely photograph of Keira, I can see why! To Joe and Loanna, thank you so much for your courageous decision and for gifting Max with the chance of a new lease of life."

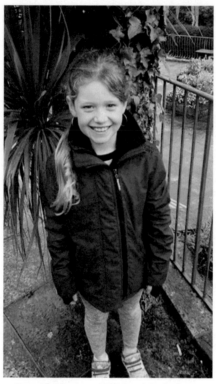

Beautiful 9-year-old Keira, Max's donor
Photo Credit: Joe and Loanna Ball

It was an emotional week away, as in that same week, we learned that the little girl whose seventh birthday party Max had been the DJ for, had lost her battle, whilst waiting for a second heart transplant. Max had formed a true friendship with this sweet child. During a walk they shared one afternoon, the children and their chaperones paused to reflect in the hospital's chapel. Sitting side by side on the pew, these two courageous youngsters prayed for one another to receive the gift of life they both so needed. Tragically, the wait for this precious wee angel was just too long. She is another child who we think of often.

Our relationship with Joe and Loanna went from strength to strength. We were consistently moved by the way they would positively comment ('like' in Facebook speak) on things involving Max, including the myriad memories which popped up, as the first anniversary of so many things – unique at this time to our situation, such as the fitting of Max's heart pump – approached.

The Ball family was also incredibly brave in sharing their story with the Mirror newspaper at a critical time in the run up to the vote in Parliament on the 23 February 2018. It was crucial that enough MPs attended to have their say and vote on the Private Member's bill – The 'Organ Donation Deemed Consent Bill'. This bill was passed without objection and we are firm in our belief that The Mirror article about Keira and Max could well have persuaded enough MPs to attend and therefore pushed the campaign over the line. For all those readers who had been following Max's journey in the news, this was the final *golden* centrepiece in his story; the identity of Max's donor.

The headline read:

'"Our little girl's heart saved Max's life": Dad of loving crash victim, 9, reveals how her organs helped four people.'

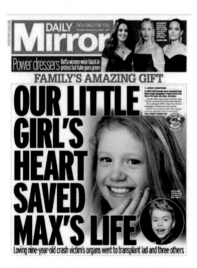

Keira on the front page of the Mirror
Photo Credit: Joe and Loanna Ball/Mirror Newspaper Group

A few days later, another article was printed, encouraging MPs to attend the 'Organ Donation Deemed Consent Bill' second reading and debate in Parliament:

'"You have the chance to save lives!" Boy, 10, with new heart begs MPs to vote to change organ donor laws.'

It was vital that a minimum of 100 MPs attended the reading, and we feel sure that the Ball family's brave decision to share their story at such a pivotal political moment may well have helped to get the Bill passed.

Emma was invited to observe the debate from within the Chamber. It was very difficult for her when the Ball family's MP stood up and recounted what had happened to Keira on that tragic day, a couple of days before Max's transplant. Emma found herself welling up with emotion and had to step out of the Chamber for a few moments. At the end of the three-hour debate, Emma said she could hear a pin drop when the question was asked whether there were any objections. Before she quite realised it, the bill was passed. The Mirror team sitting in the gallery were delighted and gave Emma a 'Thumbs Up!'. All that hard work and persistence seemed to be paying off. The previous evening, there had been a reception hosted by the Mirror. Emma was invited onto the panel to speak at the event. Also providing their experiences were Andy Cole, ex-Manchester United footballer (who had a transplanted kidney donated by his nephew), Fiona Loud (from Kidney Care UK), Kaylee-Ann Davidson-Olley (who, as a baby, had a heart transplant over thirty years ago at the Freeman Hospital), MP Jackie Doyle-Price, Secretary of State for Mental Health and Inequalities and Patricia Carroll (whose daughter, Natalie, died in 2014 awaiting a new pancreas and kidney. Patricia subsequently donated a kidney to a young man on Natalie's ward). A truly representative panel and for Emma, it was a new, surreal and quite overwhelming experience, but she managed to answer the questions with composure, honesty and candour. Keira Ball was never far from her mind. That beautiful little face, sparkling with personality.

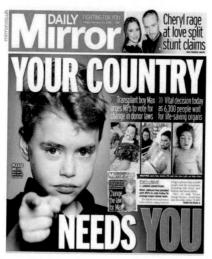

Max urging MPs to vote for change in donor law
Photo Credit: Andy Stenning/Mirror Newspaper Group

The Mirror captured that momentous day:

'From intense emotion to immense pride: How MPs made history by voting in favour of opt out organ register'

What was incredible about the debate was that support for a change to the organ donation rules had cross-party accord. This was not a party-political issue. Transplantation can affect anybody, no matter your political leanings or genetic make-up; organ failure is consistently devastating.

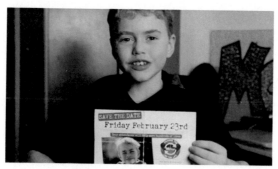

Max urging MPs to vote on the 23rd February 2017
Photo Credit: Andy Stenning/Mirror Newspaper Group

It was in May of 2018, that a date was finally set for us to meet Keira's family.

Joe and Loanna were heading to Cheshire for a family function, so they felt that the timing was perfect. It made complete sense to coincide the meeting with a planned event, rather than trying to organise something specifically. We would meet at our house on the Friday afternoon, and it was agreed that it would be a great opportunity to share the story with the Mirror; people could see the heart-warming consequences of Joe's decision to donate and what it meant to both families. All the time, we were both looking to raise awareness of organ donation, but to do so through the power of a touching human story.

Nervous doesn't cut it, as we waited for the Ball family to arrive. "Is the house tidy?" (c'mon, it never is), "I hope the food is okay?" Just relax. Forget about the garden – we relinquished that to Mother Nature months ago. All proudly wearing our 'InspiredbyKeira' tops, we waited. With a smooth one hundred and eighty degree turn, Joe landed the people carrier in the drive. "They're here" went up the shout as we lined ourselves up to greet our very special guests. Online, one can find recordings of people meeting donor families for the first time, so I guess this informs how you 'think' it will go; immediate tears and hugs. Well, our greeting was typically British! Hugs and handshakes, yes, but details about the journey over and how the hotel was, dominated the initial stages of the conversation. Somehow, it just didn't seem right to gush – I wanted the emotion, when it came, to be rooted in sincerity and appropriate.

Drinks made, we sat and continued our gentle chat for some fifteen minutes, before Emma collected the stethoscope. Provided by one of our friends for this meeting, Emma asked if anyone would like to listen to Max's heart. A not so orderly queue formed, and Max dutifully lifted his 'InspiredbyKeira' top, to reveal his scarred little chest, in which Keira's precious heart was now beating. "I can't hear it," said Katelyn – what? – no, wait, Max's red lips, pink cheeks and general lack of anything approximating oxygen deficiency confirmed that his heart simply must be beating.

"If you look between his ribs on the left, you can see it," I said. Sure enough, Max's intercostal muscles would relent in time with the beating of his wonderful little power pack of a heart.

"Ooh, it's fast," said Keely-Rose (transplanted hearts do beat faster than normal).

"In fairness, he's a little excited," I replied. When Joe heard his daughter's heart beating, his eyes filled with tears and he and Max hugged. It was the opening act of a very real bond they share to this day.

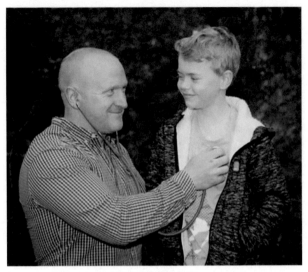

Max with Joe Ball
Photo Credit: Andy Stenning/Mirror Newspaper Group

We chatted further – learned more about the terrible incident which befell the family on that fateful day – and heard of the terrible struggle to pick up the pieces of their lives after such a devastating time. Joe talked movingly of his decision to donate Keira's organs and how, seeing ambulances taking his and Keira's little gifts to the luckiest of recipients, was the hardest thing he'd ever witnessed. One thing was clear; Joe was resolute in his belief that he had made the right choice. Why? Well, he was sure of one thing: "It's what Keira would have wanted." There, in Joe's statement was something which is at the very heart of organ donation; the wishes of the donor. Joe found courage and confidence in his unswerving belief that Keira – who would do anything to help anyone – would have wanted her Dad to donate her organs. A bright, thoughtful little girl, it was clear that Keira would have understood what her Dad was doing and would have approved.

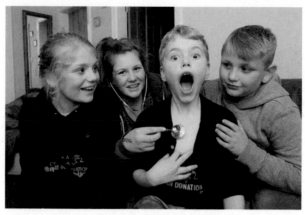
Max with Keira's siblings
Photo Credit: Andy Stenning/Mirror Newspaper Group

As the afternoon gave way to evening, Jeremy Armstrong and a photographer from the Mirror arrived (they had thoughtfully delayed their entrance), and by the side of a dwindling pile of sandwiches and cakes, we had our opportunity to say 'thank you' to Joe and Loanna for what they had done for us. Actually, 'thank you' seems wholly inadequate; how can you properly convey your sinew deep feelings of gratitude towards a family whose actions directly saved Max. The only thing you can do is speak from the heart; the time was right. We could never truly appreciate what Joe, Loanna and their family have been through. Yes, we had been through incredibly challenging times and had endured a tortuous uncertainty for too long, but in the end, and thanks to them, we had Max. However, the realisation that you cannot truly appreciate what they must be feeling comes wrapped up in one simple, yet hugely powerful word; hope.

You see, during our entire stay in hospital, we always had hope. At no stage did the medical team need to sit us down and say "We're very sorry, Emma and Paul, but there is nothing more we can do for Max." Believe me when I say, there were times when we must have come very close, and with some parents at the Freeman, that is the conversation which ultimately shatters their world. In our case, however faint that glimmer of hope became, that pinprick of light against a jet-black sky, it was never extinguished. That is the difference. Whilst you have hope, you have everything to play for. Once hope and thus the loved one who was your everything are gone, then the darkness must be all-consuming and the Herculean challenge of how to reintroduce light to your world begins. Perhaps the light can come from many different sources, one of which may be organ donation. All I can say is that it must be a slow, unforgiving process as you try to establish your lives once more, without someone who brought such joy and love to your world.

What Joe Ball did for us, was to gently, lovingly take our faint glimmer of hope and hand it to the surgeons at the Freeman, and with that most precious gift of Keira's heart, give them the chance to turn our longed-for hope into reality. That's the incredible thing people who donate bestow – the opportunity to turn hope into reality. Yes, the supremely talented surgeons need to do their part and they did – at first keeping Max strong enough for long enough to receive his gift – and then in transplanting his new heart in place of his old, failing one. Their work, however, is purely academic, without the priceless little gifts bestowed by decent people doing something remarkable. They say that, in life, you should never meet your heroes. We met ours – Joe Ball – and we were suitably humbled. What a guy.

After an emotionally draining but uplifting evening, Joe, Loanna and the kids left for much needed rest ahead of their family function the next day. We had agreed that on Sunday, they would pop round again. Max had already let it be known that he wanted to move in next door to the Ball family in Devon; something which resounded positively with Keely-Rose and Katelyn. All I had wanted, at the end of our meeting, was for Joe and Loanna to feel that their daughter's heart had gone to a good and decent little boy who would make the most of his life and to a family who would forever cherish the memory of their little princess.

Sunday panned out much as Friday had – sadly, I could not supply the southwest sauce with which Joe had been so taken on the Friday evening as he tucked in to the buffet. I did, however, manage copious cups of tea as we chatted, overlooking the wilderness which passed as our back garden. The kids entertained themselves on Harry's swegway and Max's scooter, with the girls excitedly relaying what were clearly Max's attempts to be cool in the eyes of his new friends. He's an extrovert for sure, so any chance to show off his 'cool' credentials is not to be missed; even if it can be misplaced on occasion! After several brews and the continuation of an ongoing debate between Joe and Loanna (a farming girl) about how many sheep constituted a farm, rather than merely a hobby (I was given clear instructions by Joe not to sit on the fence, so I agreed with him!), Joe, Loanna and the kids set off for the airport and the flight home to Devon.

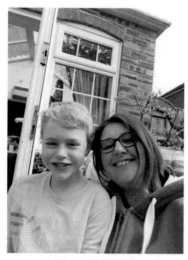

Max with Loanna
Photo Credit: Paul Johnson

The Mirror captured that first meeting beautifully:

'"Our sister's heart lives on in Max": Emotional meeting between family of tragic girl and the transplant boy whose life she saved.'

It was a poignant tribute to a very special little girl and her courageous family.

We agreed that we would keep in touch and meet again; quite possibly at the North Devon Show later in the year, where the Ball family were hoping to host an 'InspiredbyKeira' stall.

Remarkably, the North Devon Show coincided with the first anniversary of Keira's death and Max's transplant, so Emma and Max made the five-hour trip to Devon to be with the Ball family for what was going to be an emotionally charged time for them. Earlier in the book, I mentioned the nameless acts of kindness and love which characterised the reaction of people to Max's illness and his treatment. These acts have continued in many guises to this day, but one that deserves special mention actually facilitated Max and Emma's trip to Devon. Out of the blue, we were contacted by The

Leo Group, a renewable energy company from Halifax. Danny, the owner, had heard of Max's story and wanted to do something to help. With the assistance of Jasmine – one of Danny's team – they offered to provide the accommodation and meals for Max and Emma during their stay in Devon. Danny's generosity not only allowed the visit to take place; they funded a stay in a lovely hotel, which ensured that the trip to Devon was truly memorable.

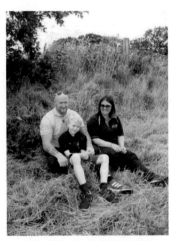

Max with Joe and Loanna at the North Devon Show 2018
Photo Credit: Emma Johnson

On the day of the show, Emma and Max joined the Ball family, members of their wider family and friends on an incredible stall, which had been beautifully bedecked in the 'InspiredbyKeira' logo. Katelyn, the younger of the two sisters, bravely agreed to have her head shaved for the Princess Trust for Wigs for children with cancer, and it was Max who was entrusted with making the first cuts. Both Emma and Max then made their way to the main arena, where they both gave a speech. Emma had originally planned to speak ahead of Max, but she was overcome with emotion after hearing Keira's Grandfather speak, so little Max stepped up to the plate, and delivered the following words;

"Hi, my name is Max and I want to say a massive thank you to the amazing Ball family. They saved my life – gave me the opportunity to do things I couldn't do – and they gave me a second chance…what more can I say. A nine-year-old girl, the beautiful Keira, died in a car crash a year ago and there will always be a dark cloud above us from that dreadful moment. I will make the most of my life, going for adventures and enjoying every minute. Keira will always be there with me. Now, I want to say 'thank you' to all of you, for supporting 'InspiredbyKeira' – it means everything to me. Thank you for listening."

Concise, as you would expect from a ten-year-old, but it said in a few words, what it needed to say and it bought Emma enough time to 'regroup'. This done, but with emotion never far from the surface, she said:

"It was some months post-transplant before we knew about Keira, but right from the start, we were acutely aware of the incredible act of kindness, generosity and humanity which gave Max his chance. Every day, whilst we watched Max grow stronger and regain the spark and energy that had been absent for so long, we wondered about our donor family and how they were coming to terms with their loss. It is the at times complex and conflicting emotions, which define transplantation; the wonderful, joyous giving of life to one, at the end of life for another. One is reassured by the thought that the act of giving the gift of life brings comfort and a feeling of warmth to a grieving family in the midst of what must be a very cold and dark time.

They say that in life, you should never meet your heroes – it always ends in disappointment. Well, let me dispel that received wisdom. We got to meet our hero, and our love and admiration for Joe and his family has only grown deeper with the passage of time. We cannot imagine the pain that Joe, Loanna, Keely-Rose, Katelyn and Bradley and their wider family and friends have felt and – I have no doubt – continue to feel for the loss of their beautiful daughter, Keira. Yet, to meet them is to meet a wonderful family, whose dignity and courage is exceptional and whose capacity to think of others, firstly with the incredible act of donating Keira's organs, but then in setting up InspiredbyKeira, is inspiring in itself. It is the most poignant and powerful representation of the goodness and strength in the human spirit.

Organ donation is so powerful, like little else – what more can one human being do for another than to save their life? Every organ donor and their families are heroes who choose to do something incredible. We are just remarkably privileged to have met our hero, Joe Ball, and his amazing family, and whilst we never met Keira, she is and always will be a part of our family. Thank you."

The following day, Emma and Max were invited to Loanna's parents' farm near Barnstaple. It was idyllic and set in the beautiful Devon countryside. Emma and Max were offered the chance to have a go at quad biking. It was thrilling, although Emma, being risk-averse, was very nervous. What really touched Emma and Max, was the 'Heartiversary' cake that Joe had designed and organised. It was red and heart-shaped with a golden heart sitting on top. Iced across the cake were the names: 'Keira' and 'Max'. It said it all – two children who had never met, forever intertwined. Emma noticed a tear in Joe's eyes as Max proudly cut the cake. Such a caring and thoughtful idea to embrace Max's special day, despite it being one year since they had lost their own child.

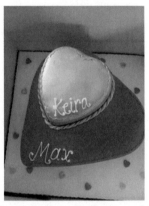

Max's 'First Heartiversary' cake, courtesy of the Ball family
Photo Credit: Emma Johnson

In one of Max's interviews for BBC North West Tonight, he was asked how it feels to have a law named after him. He looked down and quietly said, "It would be nice if the law could be called 'Max and Keira's Law.'" The change in the law, when it comes, will also be a part of Keira's mark on the world.

The evening of 29 October 2018 was – in terms of the weather – as it should have been; cold, somewhat windy and most definitely inclement. We stood in the now darkness of early evening, huddled against the cruel wind, waiting to join the red carpet which led to the 2018 Pride of Britain awards. Max had been nominated for an award and had been selected as a winner of the 'Child of Courage' category. What a contrast, we thought, to two years before as we were by this time becoming increasingly worried about our little boy's failing health. We were ushered onto the red carpet by a producer, past the phalanx of photographers, who hollered at us to 'clear the background' so they could capture a shot of some celebrity from one of the myriad reality TV shows and headed into a beautifully decorated main ball room at the Grosvenor House Hotel on London's Park Lane. As we looked across the room towards our table, we noticed the figures of Joe and Loanna Ball, already seated and awaiting the commencement of proceedings. As Max and Joe saw one another, they both jogged on a collision course as quickly as the table arrangement allowed, and engaged in a massive hug. They have such an amazing bond. It was like the platform scene from The Railway Children when the steam lifts and father and daughter are finally reunited. We were delighted that Joe and Loanna would be sharing this evening with us – not only was the award and law change campaign that had given rise to it a part of Keira's legacy; Max would simply not be here without the Ball family, so how lovely to have them there with us for this special occasion.

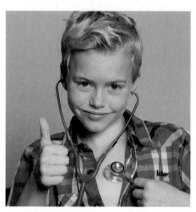

Official 'Pride of Britain' Photo
Photo Credit: Andy Stenning/Mirror Newspaper Group

Our day had started early, with a surprise for Max involving Ashely Banjo from the dance troupe 'Diversity'. We had, along with the Pride of Britain producers, conspired to surprise Max about his award on the very day of the ceremony. This was not easy to achieve – Max is a curious little fellow, and he can spot a shaky story from a mile away, so we needed to play this one cool. Emma and I had been fitted with hidden microphones at our hotel, and as we headed out into Trafalgar Square, the tall figure of Ashley Banjo was visible, just outside the National Gallery. We headed to where the famous dancer was standing, dressed in his silver suit. As we had been briefed to do, we gave Max a couple of coins, in order to get Ashley 'robot dancing'. A few robotic moves were performed, with Max actually joining in, and then Mr Banjo removed his facemask and spoke with Max. "Are you Max?"

"Yes, are you Ashley, from Diversity?" (Thank goodness Max knew who he was!)

"Yes, you know me and I know you." Max was genuinely shocked and a small crowd gathered to witness what was happening. Ashley informed Max that he would be going to the home of the Prime Minister, who had written to Max, when she decided to change the organ donation laws. Max even knew the Prime Minister's address – I was very impressed.

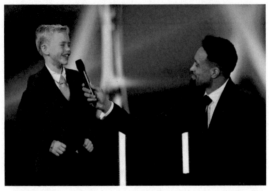

Max with Ashley Banjo on stage at The Pride of Britain Awards
Photo Credit: Andy Stenning/Mirror Newspaper Group

We arrived at 'Number 10' to be met by a wall of security; passports, driving licenses and scanners – no surprises there, then. In fairness, everything ran smoothly and we walked up Downing Street to what must be the most famous and beautifully polished front door in the world. Max rang the bell. The door was opened and we were warmly greeted by our reception team. Coats and mobile phones relinquished, we were taken on a tour of the tardis-like building. For me, the highlight was Max and Harry being allowed to sit in the Prime Minister's chair around the Cabinet table. I thought of the pre-eminent posteriors that had warmed this seat and decided that I would not want to try it for size – I felt that breaking it with my own expansive backside would be really poor form. I noticed that there were two clocks in the room; one on the mantelpiece behind where the Prime Minister sits, and one opposite, on a sideboard. We were informed that this second, sideboard clock, was placed there by Harold Wilson during his time as P.M. He had been a stickler for timekeeping, but rather than having to crane his neck to look at the mantelpiece clock, or do that thing we all do with our watches that we hope no one will notice, he had the second clock placed opposite his seating position. This simple move allowed him to run things to time, without making it look obvious that this was what he was doing. Bravo.

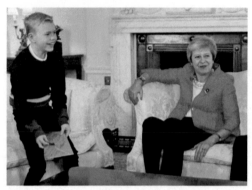

Max with Prime Minister Theresa May in The White Room of 10 Downing Street
Photo Credit: Andy Stenning/Mirror Newspaper Group

We then headed upstairs to the White Room, which is where the Prime Minister greets foreign dignitaries – those famous white chairs in front of the glorious marble fireplace. We sat and chatted, with Max and Ashley continuing their robot routine and discussing computer game strategies. It was all a tad surreal – sitting in such auspicious surroundings, flanked by cameras and chatting with Ashley Banjo about computer games. Max had just finished commenting on how amazing the chandelier was, when the Prime Minister entered the room. "You like my house, do you, Max?" asked Mrs May.

"Wow," was all Max could manage – he knew straight away with whom he was speaking and he was genuinely in awe. I couldn't have been prouder when, as the Prime Minister settled in her seat to chat with Max, he thanked Mrs May for changing the law on organ donation. Good on him, I thought, and I was glad that he did say 'thank you' – this went beyond party politics; cardiomyopathy cares not what colour rosette you wear. No, the law change was a noble act with cross party support, to help – not solve – but help the cause of awareness raising and improving consent rates. Our Prime Minister then informed Max that he would be receiving a Pride of

Britain award and handed him a gold envelope, in which was his invitation. What an amazing experience – memories with our loved ones are so important and this is one that will retain crystal clarity for the rest of our lives.

The evening itself was charged with emotion. To watch our video, filmed several weeks earlier in Cheshire under the auspices of a charity video to keep Max from guessing, was very moving. As Max went on stage to collect his award from the Leader of Her Majesty's Opposition – Mr Jeremy Corbyn – I felt a disconnect with my consciousness; it just didn't seem real or possible. Again, I felt incredibly proud of Max.

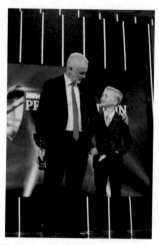

Max on stage with Jeremy Corbyn at The Pride of Britain Awards
Photo Credit: Andy Stenning/Mirror Newspaper Group

In his little speech, Max acknowledged Joe and Loanna, who thus received a spontaneous standing ovation for being the true heroes they are. Max also encouraged people to donate: "Why waste your organs, you could save four lives – nine lives." People would be forgiven for thinking Max had been prompted on what to say, but this is not the case. He knew nothing of the award in advance and he had spent many months thinking about the law change and what it meant to him. For Max, it is more of a black and white issue – why wouldn't you? – although, he fully respects people's right to choose and the reasons why it may not be so straightforward a choice. His very presence at the ceremony and the following morning on ITV's 'Lorraine' show is the most powerful representation, advocating organ donation and its transformational, lifesaving impact.

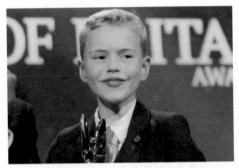

Max receiving his Child of Courage award
Photo Credit: Andy Stenning/Mirror Newspaper Group

Post awards interviews (and a 'team floss' with Jeremy Corbyn, Ashley Banjo, Olly Murs and Ellie Goulding, which set Twitter alight) over, we headed back to the hotel and collapsed into bed after a very long but thoroughly enjoyable day. It was a huge honour for Max and our family to be involved with the Pride of Britain awards, and it was humbling to see the lengths to which the organisers went, to ensure that the day was truly memorable. Max and our family have played our part in, hopefully, helping to raise awareness of organ donation, but the real heroes are those that say 'yes' when the question is asked and in so doing, save lives.

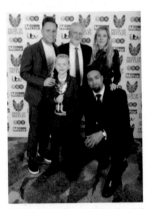

Max with Olly Murs, Jeremy Corbyn, Ellie Goulding and Ashley Banjo
who presented Max's award.
Photo Credit: Andy Stenning/Mirror Newspaper

To share the evening with Joe and Loanna seemed somehow so right. We were only there because of them. During the showing of Max's film, I looked at Loanna and could see tears in her eyes. On the screen was a picture of her beautiful daughter and I thought how her heart must yearn for that little girl every minute of every day. We have been so blessed to have been given something so utterly priceless.

At the beginning of December 2018, Emma received a message from Jeremy Armstrong at the Mirror, asking if she would be able to call the health minister's office – they needed to speak with us. Emma, whose instinct is rarely wrong, suspected what the call was about, but as she dialled the London number, she kept an open mind. Clearly, someone had been listening to Max's North West Tonight interview, where he talked of how special it would be for the law to be named 'Max and Keira's Law'. During the call, Emma was asked how we would feel about the law being named after both children in recognition of the role they had played together in this most incredible story. Emma was told that No. 10 were very keen that the idea be run past us first as a courtesy. Emma and the minister's official commented during their conversation that a number of people – including Max – had mentioned 'Max and Keira's Law', even during the debate on the floor of the House.

Emma and I had discussed a possible change to the name on a number of occasions, especially after Max himself had floated the idea. We were completely supportive of the move and were actually quite relieved that Keira's name was to join Max's; the whole story had evolved with Max and Keira now being inextricably linked. When we were first approached by the Mirror and the idea of 'Max's Law' was mooted, our son was still waiting for his transplant, hoping he would receive his second chance. Max had his little gift conferred on 2nd August and was able to continue with the campaign, providing it with a compelling and very moving insight into just what transplantation can achieve.

In the early stages of the Change the Law for Life campaign involving Max, his plight had no bearing on the fate of his donor, Keira. Their paths intertwined only because of Joe Ball and his decision to donate Keira's heart – the single most beautiful and selfless act, which makes transplantation possible. All of a sudden, the dynamic changed. Now the story unfurled to reveal the text in full; we had an utterly spellbinding case study. The change in the law relates to organ donation – how inarguably right that the beautiful little girl who gave her heart to Max be recognised for bestowing that most priceless of gifts: life itself.

In the Mirror article which announced the change, Theresa May stated: "We know more people are willing to consider organ donation than are registered donors. That is why we are changing the law to make it easier to donate – by presuming consent unless people opt out. I was reminded of the importance of this when Max visited me at No. 10. He has told of his gratitude to Keira and her family for saving his life. Her parents' courage and strength is inspiring. It's fitting we rename this important law so we can pay tribute to Keira as well as Max, to ensure her life is never forgotten."

We were four square behind the change – without Keira, it would probably still be just 'Max's Law' – goodness me, he could have the name all to himself. There is one big difference, though; it would in all likelihood be posthumous. No thank you. 'Max and Keira's Law' it is, and rightly so. On 15 March 2019, 'Max and Keira's Law' finally became official, gaining Royal Assent. A year of education and awareness raising would follow before it would be enshrined in law from spring 2020. Who would have thought it!

Since then, Joe, Loanna, Emma and Max have appeared together publicly on a couple of occasions. The first was as guest speakers at the British Transplantation Congress in Harrogate. The audience consisted of six hundred transplant professionals from the UK and beyond. Max managed to make the audience laugh, whereas Joe, Loanna and Emma had the floor in tears, such was the sadness and poignancy of their recounted experience.

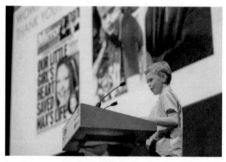

Max presenting his speech at the British Transplantation Congress 2019
Photo Credit: Andy Commins/Mirror Newspaper Group

After the event, we received a letter from Anthony Clarkson, Director of Organ Donation and Transplantation at NHS Blood and Transplant; and Stephen Wigmore, President of the British Transplantation Society, which read:

"Without reservation, the session that you participated in, along with Keira's parents, Joe and Loanna, was the most important, inspirational and impactful for all those who attended. Your presentations brought the impact on every individual and their family of waiting for an organ transplant into sharp focus. Max embodies the reason we all work in this inspiring part of the NHS, to have the chance to see him fit and well, and stealing the entire congress with his presentation was something none of us will ever forget. When combined with Keira's story, I can assure you that we all left the session inspired and determined to redouble our efforts to make every potential organ donation happen and to save the lives of every potential recipient. Once again, our heartfelt thanks for sharing your story and for all that you as a family have done to promote the importance of organ donation and transplantation across the UK."

At the congress, Max was presented with an 'Exceptional Volunteer 2019' Highly Commended Certificate in the inaugural UK awards for Excellence in Organ Donation and Transplantation. On the back of the certificate, it said:

"Max was a normal eight-year-old until he was diagnosed with dilated cardiomyopathy. He spent many difficult months in the Freeman Hospital waiting for a heart transplant. Max thankfully had his transplant carried out in August 2017 after which he made a steady recovery. As a result of their experiences, Max and his family made it their mission to raise public awareness about organ donation and the desperate shortage of donor organs and tissue in order to help others. Max's family knew from first-hand experience that his survival was entirely dependent upon the generosity of another family agreeing to organ donation. Max campaigned extensively in the media to raise awareness and for people to sign the Organ Donor Register. He featured in a powerful BBC documentary 'Heart Transplant – A Chance to Live' which generated a huge public response. His efforts to bring in an 'opt out' organ donation system in England have brought about a change to the legislation covering organ and tissue donation. A private members' bill was passed unopposed in the Commons and will introduce presumed consent for organ donors in England which has become known as 'Max and Keira's Law'. The efforts of Max and his family have had a phenomenal impact and will hopefully benefit others awaiting transplantation."

What an honour. The other occasion that saw Max, Emma, Joe and Loanna appear publicly was on the *This Morning* sofa in the early spring of 2019 for an interview with Phillip Schofield and Holly Willoughby. A nerve-wracking experience for all, but the courage of Joe and Loanna in talking about what had happened to Keira was remarkable. We are eternally grateful to them, not purely because of the precious gift that was bestowed on Max by Keira, with Joe Ball's blessing, but also for the courageous work that they continue to undertake in raising awareness about the importance of organ donation and transplantation. Thank you, Keira, and God Bless.

"To Keira,
You didn't just give Max your heart
You freed Max from pain
You gave Max a life
You gave Max a future
You gave Max love
You gave Max laughter
You gave us our child
You gave Harry his brother
You gave parents their grandson
You gave brothers their nephew
You gave schoolmates their friend
You gave teachers their pupil
You gave hope to others…The ripples run far and wide"

Emma Johnson

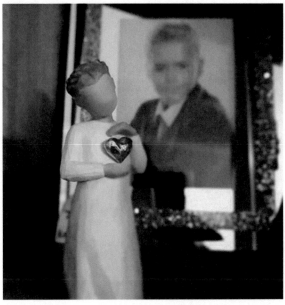

Willow Tree Keepsake Girl Figurine with Max in the Background
Photo Credit: Joe Ball

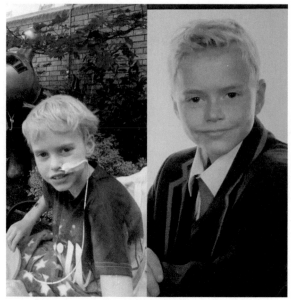

Max at his sickest on left and Max's school photo taken October 2018 on right.
Photo Credit: Emma Johnson/Academy Photography

'Conclusion'

How do you write a conclusion, to something which is ongoing? In our meeting with Dr Reinhardt in January 2017, she said to us that transplantation is a lifelong commitment; it is something that not everyone can cope with. At the time, you will do anything it takes to save your child and the idea of saying 'no' is a complete anathema. That said, there is no denying that our lives are now on a very different trajectory and as people, the seismic impact of the last few years has changed us. Whether it's your ability to cope in certain situations, or how you seek refuge from the reality you are facing, this sort of trauma taps further and deeper into your core than those challenges, which used to cause such angst.

Against a plotline of uncertainty and chronic stress, we have been privileged to meet some incredible people, who have empathised, supported and helped us along the way.

One can only speak as one finds. For nine months, our son was kept alive and ultimately given a second chance by the world-beating institution that is our National Health Service. To read of parents in other countries with children in exactly the same predicament as Max, but whose health service, such as it is, does not entertain paediatric transplantation is to witness desperation in its most crushing, painful and cruel form. To read an advice leaflet about paediatric transplantation from the wealthiest country on the planet, which tells parents how to go about funding their child's transplant, is to appreciate just how very, very lucky we have been. We will never be able to repay the NHS – indeed, we couldn't repay it in five lifetimes. Mercifully, what happened to Max is very rare, but our NHS was there for him and our family. And what of the staff we met? Extraordinary people who go to work every day and strive to do something remarkable for their patients. They are dedicated professionals who do everything clinically possible – whilst continually raising the bar – to turn the hopes of desperately anxious parents into reality. All one had to do is look at the pain and sadness on their faces when a patient didn't make it to realise that theirs is a vocation from which emotion and caring simply cannot be separated. Whatever the future delivers for Max, our family will hold a love and gratitude for the people who made his second chance possible.

I would like to share a letter that was sent to Emma and me towards the end of June 2017, by Sue, the lead psychologist on the team from whom we received so much support. Our time with Sue and her colleague, Kathryn, was central to us being able to get through the chronic stress of our situation. As you read the letter, I am sure you will appreciate that it moved us greatly.

"Dear Paul and Emma,

These last six months since Max became ill have been phenomenally challenging for you all as a family. This can't be stated strongly enough. I have been very impressed with the courage and resilience you have both shown. I admire the way you have dealt with the very significant threats that Max's illness has brought. I know there have been, and continue to be, times when the pressure feels unbearable. Yet you find strength to follow the goal of making sure Max is looked after with love, kindness, empathy and understanding. I am certain that the support you give him enables him to get through each day whilst he waits for a new heart. I try to but can't imagine the pain you both feel for Max, for yourselves and for Harry. The loss of your ordinary and carefree family life must feel so devastating. It is humbling to watch you struggle but to ultimately succeed in the ongoing battle."

In that beautiful, thoughtful letter, Sue captures the essence of our experience; being surrounded daily by such care, understanding and compassion gave rise to a relationship of profound mutual respect. I guess it boils down to a simple maxim; do unto others as you would have them do unto you. Our love for Max translated into a complete dedication to his care and a determination to play our part, alongside the professionals, in getting him over the line. To have this recognised by Sue in such a way meant a great deal to us.

Sue's letter evoked memories of a Banksy mural painted on the Heart Ward wall, in which the silhouette of a girl, hair blowing in the wind, is reaching out to grab the end of a trailing string, which is tied to a red, heart shaped balloon, blowing away. I found it such an incredibly powerful image – a metaphor for where we were – so near and yet we may as well have been a million miles away; cut adrift from the carefree life we had known – that heart floating away from the little girl captured the pain of loss, with the close yet somehow elusive reassurance of hope.

To become involved in the Mirror campaign to Change the Law for Life was certainly counter-intuitive at such a challenging time for us as a family. Whilst we have covered our rationale elsewhere, there is an additional driver behind our involvement. When we said yes to journalist, Jeremy Armstrong, with Max's full blessing, we didn't know how things were going to pan out. We didn't know if we were going to be lucky and live out the ending we dreamed of, or whether we would be saying goodbye to our little boy in Newcastle. We have always brought our sons up with the mind-set that to help others is a good thing, just as our parents had taught us. If Max could do something in his life to help others, then his time on this earth would not have been in vain. If he made it home with us as we prayed, then we could share in the warmth that doing a good deed brings. If we were to say goodbye, then at least we could look back with pride that he had done something very special in his all too short life. The Mirror team wrote, thanking us for our support:

"Just wanted to say thank you so much for everything you did to help with our campaign – today is an enormous victory. We hope you and Max and your entire family feel very proud that your courageous decision to go public when you did, may help people stay alive in the future. Thank you so much…"

Alison Phillips, Editor of the Mirror.

In return, people have been so generous in acknowledging Max's role in the campaign, with the Prime Minister stating that Max's story had inspired her decision to change the law, describing him as 'a very brave little boy' – the kindness of others is simply humbling.

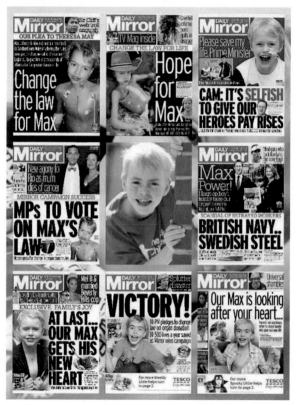

Max with some of the Mirror front pages, compiled by Roger Johnson
Photo Credit: Andy Commins/Andy Stenning/Mirror Newspaper Group

We were told, right from the start, that transplantation is not a cure – far from it. To truly get it and realise how lucky you are to have a second chance, one has to remind oneself what the alternative is. By doing this, you not only appreciate the magical, selfless humanity of someone making the decision to donate; you are in awe of the staggering complexity and progress of medical science that has made it possible.

As the parent of a transplanted child, you feel an overwhelming sense of responsibility; worry about the future and a profoundly deep sense of gratitude. This gratitude is like a star burst, touching so much. For a start, you are very lucky…yes, really. Are we lucky to have been hit with Max's illness? No, of course not, there was nothing lucky about that. However, you then have to, once again, remind yourself of the reality of the situation you face; without a transplant he will die. Max was extremely lucky that he received his gift in time. There were children on the ward who were not blessed with the same good fortune. We got to take Max home in the car at the end of his time at the Freeman Hospital – there were parents who did not get that seemingly simple, beautiful outcome. Children Max had spoken with and become friends with were called to heaven way ahead of what should have been their time. I will not name the children, suffice to say that each one of them is represented by a pure, brilliant star – a beacon showing their eternal spirit – which burns brightly in the night sky. They touched us all. They will never be forgotten.

Transplantation in many ways reminds me of the film 'AI' from 2001, in which a robot child called David is programmed with the ability to love. Set in a future where global warming has wreaked havoc on the climate, David becomes tragically parted from his adoptive human mother, whom he loves dearly. After some two thousand years in stasis, David is rescued by highly advanced robots which inhabit the earth, recognising him as the last 'living' link with human kind, now extinct. Using a lock of his mother's hair, which David had kept, his rescuers are able to bring her back to life. However, there is a caveat; they are only able to do this once, and his mother will only live for a day. Deciding to take the chance they offered, during that day, David enjoyed every second with his mother, making memories to last him a lifetime. Towards the end of their time together, before she slipped away, she confirmed to David that she had always loved him; just what he had so desperately yearned to hear. As the sun set, they lay on the bed together.

For me, this scene encapsulates the emotional, beautiful and relatively ephemeral nature of a life post-transplantation. One does not like to dwell on mortality. In life, one seeks as far as one can to accentuate the positive, but diminished life expectancy is an inescapable reality in transplantation that, as the parent of a transplanted child, is impossible to ignore. As in the scene from 'AI', in twenty-first century transplantation, cutting edge technology plays such a pivotal role; that it offers something undeniably remarkable, but one cannot be emotionally impervious to its current limitations.

Perhaps, accentuating that all-important positive, it is better viewed from the following perspective: transplantation has developed due to the pioneering work of individuals, teams of professionals and the support of charities such as the British Heart

Foundation. It has become an incredible, hard to comprehend treatment option for those for whom there is no other option. It offers hope where, in reality, there should be none. So, when a transplant takes place and the recipient is able to return home and live with their loved ones, then David's example stands true; enjoy every minute of something truly special.

When my mother passed away, she said she would save a place in heaven next to her for my father. It is warming and uplifting to think that we may indeed meet again, after our corporeal existence comes to an end, but I don't know if this is true. It may be that when we close our eyes for the last time, that's it. Ultimately, we live on ostensibly in the hearts and memories of our loved ones and those we have touched. It is what we do when we are here – the ripples we make on the pond, *whenever* we make them – that count. For Max in his short life, he has made some very real ripples and left an indelible mark on the hearts of many he has met, as has Keira. Those who make the courageous decision to donate do likewise. It is our hope that he is given the chance to make many more ripples and live a long, healthy and happy life with Keira's heart beating in his chest. One thing is for sure, we never miss an opportunity to tell him just how much we love him.

To meet the family of the little girl who saved our son's life was the most humbling experience of our lives. Max is only here today because of the decision made by Joe Ball to donate the organs of his daughter, Keira. As a family, their unimaginable suffering is beyond doubt, yet they manage to think of others through their charity 'InspiredbyKeira'. As families, we are both trying to move on with our lives, but we share an unbreakable bond, forged by Joe's utterly selfless, courageous decision to donate. Keira is a part of our family, as Max is now a part of the Ball family.

As Joe and Loanna said to us: "Life fails to be perfect, but it never fails to be beautiful."

Perhaps I should leave the last words to Max. In November 2017, he typed this recollection of his experience. Concisely written, it captures in a few short paragraphs the chronology and personal impact of a story, which reverberates widely and touches many.

"My Time in Hospital: One night, my life was about to change forever... I felt sick, faint, I couldn't breathe, my tummy was aching and my head was pounding. Dad called 111 and they immediately sent an ambulance. After a night at Leighton Hospital and a month at the Royal Manchester Children's Hospital, I was transferred to the Freeman Hospital in Newcastle. This is the drama.

I was told that my heart was too big, which is a condition called dilated cardiomyopathy. The ward I was on was filled with very sick babies, who cried non-stop. I couldn't get much rest! The nurses like Faye and Sophie were lots of fun. Faye used to have water fights with me and Sophie took me on fun walks. They were really kind.

In February, I had open-heart surgery to have a pump fitted. It saved my life! The pump went inside my chest. Its job was to pump blood around my body as my heart was only doing 15% of what it needed to do.

On the ward, I played fun games with the play ladies and watched movies. My favourite movie was the new *Jungle Book*, which we watched with the volume full blast! My best friend was called Dylan – we watched movies together.

On the 2/8/17, I GOT A NEW HEART! When I woke up, I felt better than I thought I would. I was in PICU in a cubicle.

Leaving the hospital a few weeks after my transplant was hard, but it was amazing to go home. My newly decorated room was epic. My bro was very happy to see me.

THANK YOU, EVERYONE!"

Golden Heart

"Wires, tubes, machines, heartache
Helpless, tired…'need a break'
Spirit, love, hope, fears
Laughs, burdens, regrets, tears
Babies crying, babies dying
Children sighing, children flying
Screams, beeps, corridor walking
Doctors, nurses, constant talking
Faces staring, parents sharing
Normality yearning, little ones learning
Cappuccinos, 'chocolate sprinkles'
Pressure mounts, heightened wrinkles
Brilliant stars…Angel Keira
Say a prayer…heaven's nearer!"

Emma Johnson

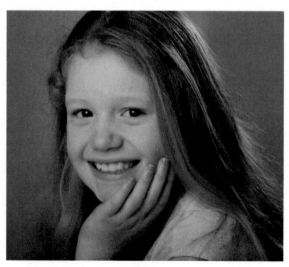

Keira

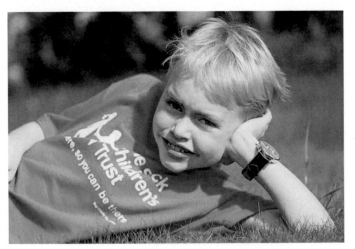

Max in the Scott House Garden, post-transplant
Photo Credit: Andy Commins/Mirror Newspaper Group

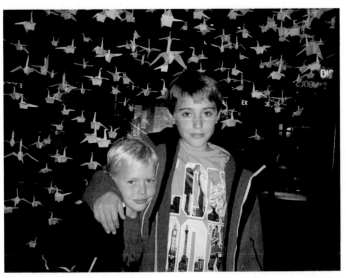

Two loving brothers, with Japanese peace cranes, before Max fell ill
Photo Credit: Marcus Taylor